READ WHAT SOME OF MY STUDENTS HAVE TO SAY ABOUT SMART DOUBLES®

*I love the consistent reminder in Ron's Smart Doubles®
program to play my location. It programs me to play smart
and use high percentage shots such as;*
Deep to Deep, Short to Short, Wide to Wide and Money Middle.
– Joey J., student, Atlanta, GA

*As someone who started playing in my 50's, Smart Doubles®
has provided a simple, common-sense way to execute doubles
strategy. I am better equipped to play smarter doubles in my
competitive league matches. "**What is Your Plan Fran**" and
"**High You Die**" are two of my favorite riffs to be more
intentional than just hitting the ball.*
– Brenda S., student, Longboat Key, Florida

*I have taken "Three and Me" clinics with Ron for several
years. With three players and the pro, it is easier to see,
understand and apply your simple, fun phrases. Ron's Riffs
are great in-the-moment shorthand reminders of smart
choices for both shot making and positioning.*
– Katie C., student, Longboat Key, Florida

Thank you, Ron for converting me into a confident, competent doubles player. I am forever grateful.
— Cynthia G., student, Sarasota, Florida

*I love your "**Sweet Roll**" riff related to a "**Short to Short**" return or defending against incoming returners or servers.*
— Stacey A., Sarasota, Florida

Smart Doubles®

Learn How to Play and Reinforce a Simple and Strategic
Game of Recreational Doubles.

Smart Doubles®
– Learn How to Play and Reinforce a Simple and Strategic Game of Recreational Doubles

F I R S T   E D I T I O N
Published in 2023 by
SMART DOUBLES LLC

ISBN: 979-8-9886023-0-9

Library of Congress Control
Shields, Ronald
Smart Doubles *– Learn How to Play and Reinforce a Simple and Strategic Game of Recreational Doubles*
Control Number: 1-12687370171 June, 2023

Category: Sports & Recreation, Tennis, Coaching, Instruction
Written by: Ron Shields | www.SmartDoubles.com | Fla10Spro@aol.com
Chief Editor: Stacey Wilson | info@TheWritingProfessor.com
Cover Designed & Formatted by: Eli Blyden Sr. | EliTheBookGuy.com
Inside Photos and Back Cover Photo by: Brenda Shields
Printed and Published in the USA: Tampa Bay, Florida

IN MEMORY

STEVE CHRISTIAN
First Tennis Coach
October 23, 1953- August 15, 1988

* *

TANNER "TEE" GARY
Nephew and Designer of Smart Doubles Trademark and Logo
August 8, 1972- February 22, 2020

* * *

DISCLAIMER

The information in this book is meant to supplement, not replace, proper (tennis) training. Like any sport involving speed, equipment, balance and environmental factors, (tennis) poses some inherent risk. The author and publisher advise readers to take full responsibility for their safety and know their limits. Before practicing the skills described in this book, be sure that your equipment is well maintained, and do not take risks beyond your level of experience, aptitude, training, and comfort level.

The reader should regularly consult a physician in matters relating to his/her health and particularly with respect to any symptoms that may require diagnosis or medical attention.

This book is not intended as a substitute for the medical advice of physicians. Before practicing the skills described in this book, be sure to consult with a physician.

PREFACE

In theory, playing and enjoying tennis can be for everyone. One intent for authoring this book is to make the social game of doubles easier to learn, play, and enjoy for a larger population of potential recreational players. If you currently do not play tennis, I hope this book will inspire and encourage you to learn, practice, enjoy, and benefit from tennis through the fun, social game of doubles. If you currently play tennis for recreation, I hope this book about doubles will enhance your success and enjoyment of tennis.

At the end of certain chapters, I have provided a blank page for your notes and questions. Perhaps, you may want to document your intentions, journey, and growth as a recreational doubles player. After your matches, clinics, or practice sessions, you may wish to make notes about how you plan to use or implement any aspect of Smart Doubles®. For example, you may want to record your plan to keep more balls in play when in a deep position or near the baseline or how you will finish more points at net with good position.

Thank you for purchasing my book. I hope you benefit greatly and share with other players.

SMART DOUBLES

CONTENTS

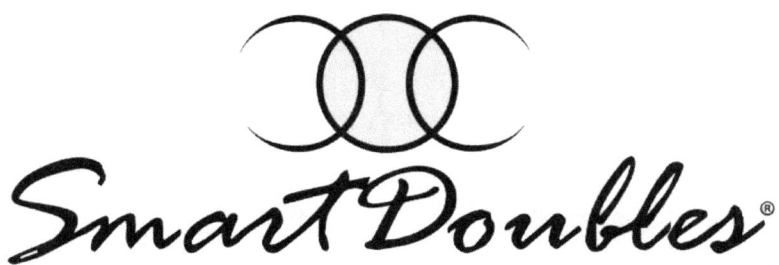

SmartDoubles®

Learn How to Play and Reinforce a Simple and Strategic
Game of Recreational Doubles.

by RON SHIELDS

SMART DOUBLES

INTRODUCTION

The main purpose for authoring this book about doubles is to help make it feasible for more people to learn, play, and enjoy doubles as a regular, life-long physical activity.

D oubles play often comes with new friends, new experiences, regular exercise, growth opportunities, and many enjoyable positive benefits and memories. After all, based on recent research you should live 9.7 years longer if you play tennis compared to other physical activities according to the Copenhagen Heart Study.[8] This research was published in the September 4th Mayo Clinic Proceedings in 2018. It indicates incredibly positive benefits to playing tennis and especially doubles given its social nature that makes people feel connected. There is consistent and credible research that proves an active lifestyle that includes regular exercise and physical activity in the spirit of fun helps to prevent, correct, and improve the conditions for many people with chronic diseases.

Another important reason for authoring this book about Smart Doubles® is to provide a straightforward approach for new, current, and returning players to learn, improve, and excel at playing a quality, strategic and fun game of recreational doubles. In other words, in the book, I teach you how to play

Smart Doubles®, how to improve your current play, how to win more matches, and how to enjoy and benefit from the game of doubles. Also, I seek to equip and encourage other teaching professionals, coaches, and public and private facility managers to teach, implement, and promote Smart Doubles® clinics and related events for both juniors and adults. Those who currently play or want to play doubles should seek to learn and play Smart Doubles®!

In my view, pickleball and other paddle games have become increasingly popular because too many tennis courts are simply idle waiting for players or an instructor to appear to provide clinics or events. In many cases, public hard courts are taken over by pickleball. This court idleness makes it easy for public and private managers/owners to paint and stripe existing tennis courts for pickleball activity as a tennis alternative. However, many players enjoy both sports. Personally, I see ping pong or table tennis as the perfect tennis alternative or substitute which can be played with soft or hard paddles, larger or smaller balls, indoors or outdoors, and on various softer surfaces with little formal instruction! It is good exercise, fun, and stimulating with NO kitchen to get burned in. Also, playing table tennis will improve your hand-eye coordination that will make it easier to enjoy other sports including tennis. For the record, the best exercise or activity is the one that you enjoy and will do regularly.

I will acknowledge that tennis mechanics and strokes are more technical and require more patience, work, and practice for most people to master. In addition, private tennis lessons can be expensive depending on the area, location, facility, and instructor. Also, the competitive game of singles requires more fitness, athleticism, practice, and proficiency of skills compared to other racquet/paddle sports. Therefore, a game like pickleball or table tennis is much easier for many to simply get started and enjoy without a significant investment of money, time, or physical exertion on a much smaller area of play. However, tennis, especially doubles, offers a more robust package of benefits, especially long-term once you learn how to stroke the ball and return the ball somewhat consistently and play.

Many of us witnessed via television the 2022 US Open where several top ranked professional athletes played four sets of singles for over three hours. Before the finals, 19-year-old Alcaraz had to recover from beating Sinner and Tiafoe in five grueling sets in each match. In my view, these top 100 elite professional tennis players are the fittest athletes among all sports. However, this book is not about this relatively small group of professional-level tennis players. It is about the majority, not the minority, of the total population who want to learn to play or resume playing, and those who currently play. These are the recreational tennis players who play for fun, physical activity, and comradery among other active people in their community. It is estimated by the most recent International Tennis Federation's Global Participation Report published in 2021, that approximately eighty-seven million people, or 1.71% of the population participated in tennis at least once during a 12-month period during 2020.[7] This report surveyed forty-one national tennis organizations that make up 90% of total players, coaches, clubs, and courts in the world.[7] China (22.9%), the US (24.8%) and India (10.2%) combined account for just more than 55% of the global tennis population.[7]

Also, from this report there are 585 players for every coach with an estimated 149,110k certified coaches with 59% of these coaches being based in Europe. In addition, the USA owns the most courts by nation estimated at 37% with China in second place at 8.6%. The estimation of total tennis courts is 589k according to this report.[7]

According to statistical research conducted by the Physical Activity Council (PAC Study) in 2020 for the Tennis Industry Association, reported in 2021 approximately 21.64 million players in the USA.[11] From this study, there is a core group of 11.63 million who plays more frequently ten or more times per year.[11] In addition to this core group (frequent, regular, avid), there is a significant non-core group of players that range from occasional and casual participation to people thinking about playing in the future. The 2021 TIA report as well as the 2019 report reflect 71% and 73% of total players are 18+ years of age.[11] Also, it is particularly challenging to determine how many tennis instructors there are in the USA who are working part-time, full-time, certified, or not certified. My guess is that there is a shortage of working tennis instructors relative to the total number of current and prospective players in the USA.

Based on my general analysis of two ITF reports and several TIA reports, it seems there are millions of interested people all over the world who are excellent candidates to begin playing again (especially in the 25-44 age group), or to learn how to play, mix, mingle, and enjoy tennis as beginners to intermediate players. It is particularly challenging to determine accurately how many people are interested in playing tennis, how many do play tennis, how many times and where exactly, and specific levels at which they play; unless they play competitively or "belong" to a club, facility or organization that is tracking and willing to share the correct information. From my fifty plus years of being around tennis, it seems that most recreational players play tennis occasionally or seasonally for fun, social, and exercise, not for rankings or more serious competition such as leagues and tournaments. In general, spring, summer, and fall are prime times for most players in most areas to enjoy tennis. Thanks to the internet, we can locate some, not all, courts, programs, clinics, players, and teaching professionals online through various apps and websites. It is my belief, that if more core players (avid, regular, weekly) and non-core players (occasional, casual, procrastinators) better understood and enjoyed the game of doubles the more occasions (leagues, ladders, clinics, mixers, round robins, social games) they would participate in on a regular basis.

Many current and regular players do not have a court access problem. But many do have a challenge finding courts depending on the time of the year or where they live. In addition, many people even with good court access may play infrequently or not at all for distinct reasons while others struggle to find both courts and people with whom to play. Common sense says why, when, and how often people play tennis depends on their location-access, time of the year, and available players for the opportunity to play. Friends, family, and peer pressure may or may not be a motivating factor for the why to play tennis. Those who live in warmer climates may be able to play with good court access close to year-round while those who live in colder and indoor tennis markets will struggle for court availability. As you can imagine, indoor court time is more expensive than outdoor courts. Often outdoor courts are free or low-cost. During the spring, summer and fall mostly, as a kid and teen, I was able to ride my bike or walk to play outdoors on public courts. Also, in my hometown, there was little to no junior program access with instruction in the public sector. Indoor court time for playing as a kid/teen during winter months was rarely an option for me.

Depending on where you live and your resources, you may or may not have access to courts, instructors, clinics, and leagues. Therefore, access to play and learn tennis is driven by your public sector- parks, schools, community courts, or your private sector- private clubs. Often the private sector is the only or best game in town. Unfortunately, in many areas the public courts are in disrepair or demolished making it challenging to impossible for their community to learn and enjoy tennis. However, many municipalities do a fantastic job providing public and community courts. If you have access to public courts use them before they disappear! During the Covid 19 Pandemic many people became keenly aware that playing tennis outdoors was an excellent option for physical activity and social distancing! News Flash- before the Covid 19 Pandemic playing tennis outdoors was a win-win for the general population. Another attractive feature and benefit to playing tennis is its socially connecting nature making it a healthier activity compared to other activities done alone such as going to the gym, swimming, or cycling.

With this book, I am promoting doubles, specifically, Smart Doubles®, as a way for more people to benefit and enjoy holistically recreational tennis at various levels and abilities. To begin your journey at enjoying the game of doubles even in a casual or fun context, you only need three -four players and a court. Just go out and hit the ball around with an underhand, drop hit or regular overhead serve. However, if feasible, I recommend small group lessons/clinics (three -six players) at a much lower cost per person especially for beginners, advanced beginners, and intermediate players to learn and reinforce good stroke mechanics, fundamentals, and consistency. In chapter 12, I will recommend alternative ways to improve your strokes and specific shot making if access to a good coach/programming is not feasible or convenient. As a reminder, this is not an instructional book about your biomechanics and strokes. It is about the basic strategy and proper positioning of playing doubles, being more successful at doubles play, and enjoying doubles for fun and recreation. You do not have to hit the ball hard or fast like a pro to enjoy playing doubles at your current level. Why you play tennis is personal, and how you benefit from playing tennis is also personal. Through my Smart Doubles® program, I seek to help more players maximize their enjoyment of tennis through the game of doubles.

Nowadays, there are several quality online teachers, videos, and instructional books that provide convenient basic tips and instruction at a lower cost for improving strokes and technique. Tennis can be expensive to learn and play, especially on a private lesson and private club basis. A popular perception is that tennis is expensive, exclusive, and too complicated related to access to courts, lessons, programs, and proper equipment. The reality is tennis equipment such as balls can range from $3 to 6 dollars per can, and good, adequate new or used racquets can be purchased from $50 to 100 per racquet. Yes, racquets come in varied sizes, shapes, weights, lengths, and they will eventually need new strings and grips. It is important that you demo a few racquets and eventually buy a good racquet that is right for you, your level and budget. Your hands grip the racquet, but your strings feel and grip the ball. In a recent conversation with Sammy Aviles, (former colleague at the Colony Beach & Tennis Resort and Longboat Key Club), I realized that strings are like tires. A good racquet with bad strings is the same as a good car with bad tires. Both can cause accidents. Be knowledgeable of your strings and tension options.

Of course, you can always pay more for anything tennis related if you like based on your budget and shopping preferences. However, there are online resources, teaching pros, tennis shops, and players willing to guide you with your personal equipment. Regarding learning how to play or improve, sharing the costs to play doubles or taking small group clinics is a more affordable approach to tennis and perhaps more fun too than most people think. In addition, according to an article published in September 2019 online by the National Recreation and Parks Association, most of the tennis play in the U.S., at least 70%, takes place on public courts that are free or at low costs.[9] Unless you are seeking to be a tennis professional, or collegiate tennis player, the cost and time to be a good recreational doubles player can be reduced by using several low- cost, self-enhancing tools including this book and other tools to be discussed.

If you currently play doubles or would like to learn or improve at doubles, wouldn't you prefer to play "Smart Doubles"! In this book, I will share my program and experience at teaching and coaching Smart Doubles®. As a teaching professional for 30 plus years, I wish to inspire and create smarter players and play than "not so smart" or "dumb doubles" play and players. Who is Smart Doubles® for? Anyone willing to learn and play doubles. In addition, I am seeking other enthusiastic teaching professionals to become Smart Doubles® affiliates to teach, promote and reinforce Smart Doubles® at your facility or in your community to your recreational doubles players. It seems that most 18+ adults who play recreational tennis, even if they prefer singles, play and enjoy doubles too. As a tennis player and enthusiast, you are likely very entertained and in awe of certain young and popular professional singles players at certain tournament matches on television. However, it seems most tennis players between 2.5-4.5 NTRP levels (advanced beginner to advanced) play recreational doubles for fun, social, and physical activity in or near their residential community. Many current players are self-taught or informally taught by a spouse, friend, or a more advanced player. Access to courts alone does not equip and empower prospective and current players to enjoy and fully benefit from the game.

I authored this book to reach and positively impact a large population of potential and current recreational players. The Smart Doubles® program seeks to encourage, enable, and equip these players at various levels to obtain more enjoyment and success now at playing doubles. As teaching professionals, instructors, coaches, and even advanced players, we teach and coach players as well as direct them to the recreational arena in which they can learn, grow, and excel. We have the skills and ability to "grow the game" through the correct programming. Doubles strategy and positioning is more challenging to learn and apply when players and partners have a different approach, opinion, or philosophy for distinct reasons. Simplicity and common sense are key components of Smart Doubles®. Teaching professionals and programs that feature, promote, and implement Smart Doubles® will enable more recreational players to efficiently and effectively learn how to play and enjoy doubles. Singles- two players- is a terrific way to enjoy tennis, but doubles-four players- is twice the fun!

GLOSSARY OF IMPORTANT TERMS

As you may know, the language of tennis can be involved and complicated. In the book, I have created a glossary of important terms for your reference and understanding. These terms are consistently used throughout the book, and many will be abbreviated for simplicity.

NTRP: Rating system that outlines and describes characteristics of various levels from beginner (1.5) through touring pro (7.0). This rating system is commonly used in U.S. based leagues and USTA tournaments.

UTR: Universal Tennis Rating that describes level ranges for men and women individually from 1.0 to 16.5 based on actual match results.

Recreational Player: One who plays mostly for fun and recreation. Their level of skill is measured in the middle of the rating systems such as 2.5-4.5 on NTRP or 2.0-6.5 on UTR. Another way to describe a recreational player is to generally classify them as an advanced beginner, intermediate, advanced intermediate, or an advanced player. For comparison, collegiate and professional level players are rated at the top end of the rating systems. These more advanced players are rated from 5.0-7.0 on NTRP and 8.0-16.5 on UTR.

Mechanics/Strokes: The technical details of how to strike or hit the ball related to grip, hand, racquet face, arm, backswing, contact, follow through, feet or stance, and balance or weight transfer.

Groundstrokes: After the ball bounces you hit forehands and backhands.

FH: Forehand groundstroke.

BH: Backhand groundstroke.

Serve: Refers to toss above head and striking the ball above the server's head. Also, informally, can mean to drop hit or underhand strike to start a point.

T Serve: Small area in either service box that is divided by the vertical center line. Also known as serving up the middle and near the vertical line.

Volley: Describes a ball or shot that is hit with no bounce out of the air in transition to the net or at the net.

Overhead: This stroke will be described as an OH. The overhead is a stroke like the serve that is hit out of the air usually hit near the net. It is also called the overhead smash. An overhead is hit in response to a lob.

Shot: Describes where and how the ball goes such as a cross court, down the line, down the middle, high, low, flat, lob, into the net etc.

Contact Zone/Area: This term refers to where you contact the ball in relation to your body and balance. There are early, perfect, comfortable, and late contact areas. Another way to discuss contact is spacing between you and the ball.

Strike Point: Where your sweet spot area or your racquet strings connect with the ball.

CC: Cross court.

DTL: Down the line.

Server: The person who serves from the baseline to start a rally, point, or game; S.

Server's Partner: The partner of the server who is positioned at the net or baseline; SP.

Returner: The person receiving the serve; R

Returner's Partner: The player not receiving the serve who is usually positioned at the service line or baseline line; RP.

NML: No Man's Land. The large area midway between the service line and baseline.

At the Net: In a position to volley or hit overheads at the service line or closer to the net as halfway between the net and service line.

High Percentage Shot: The best or smartest shot or shot options to hit based on the player's location/situation to either maintain a rally, set up, or finish the point.

Poaching: Intercepting an anticipated CC shot by moving to the right or left (across or towards the center line) to attack with a FH or BH volley.

Teaching: Technical learning, demonstrating and development of how to hit or stroke the ball as in the serve, forehand, backhand, volley and overhead. Teachers provide information and instruction.

Coaching: Showing students how, when, where and why to implement and execute specific ways, shots, and tactics to win such as playing smart, consistent, hitting to opponent's backhand or body, and maintaining a good attitude. We coach, motivate, and inspire students.

Tennis Professional: Trained and certified who coaches and teaches.

Dumb Doubles: The opposite of Smart Doubles®. Being in the wrong or an awkward location/position that does not support your partner's efforts and shots. Hitting risky shots or trying to win the point when out of position or struggling. Not being patient and overhitting thus making too many unnecessary unforced errors. Little to no communication between partners about how to support and complement each other to create and enjoy more success during a match or game.

CHAPTER 1

WHAT IS SMART DOUBLES®

S mart Doubles® is my registered trademark and evidence-based teaching/learning program for recreational players. To enjoy and be more successful at playing doubles you want to hit more *high- percentage shots* based on your location/position and always be in the best position/location as much as possible to either set up, defend, or finish the point. A *high percentage* shot is a **smart shot** that serves a purpose. It could be a deep cross court backhand hit from a deep location from your baseline area to keep the rally going or an overhead smash or volley hit to the middle between two players to finish the point. *Simply, Smart Doubles® features a strategic, purposeful, and competitive game of recreational doubles designed to create more fun, success, and growth.*

We can only hear and absorb so much in-person instruction for certain reasons. My hope is that regardless of age and level of play as a recreational player, you will benefit from this simple and common-sense presentation of Smart Doubles®. In this book, I define a recreational player as someone who wants to learn and play doubles or is currently playing doubles at a 2.5-4.5 NTRP level. Also, you can be a self-rated player (beginner, advanced beginner, intermediate, advanced) based on your experience and benefit from this book. You can learn more about ratings at the USTA's website or UTR's (Universal Tennis Rating) website for a full description of the various levels. Regardless of rating, knowing where to be, what to do and your role will help you learn and improve at doubles. Learning, reinforcing, and creating good habits of playing Smart Doubles® can be improved and developed through this book.

This book does not cover EVERY *situation* that could take place in recreational doubles play nor does it focus on professional players or a professional level of performance. However, in general, it does provide a foundation for strategic Smart Doubles® and depicts the most recurring *situations* that will occur based on two people on the same side of the net playing against two others on the other side of the net in three specific *formations*. What makes doubles unique is the simple fact of two people positioned somewhere on each side of the net! Therefore, the game of doubles can be simplified based on the limited and predictable *situations* that can occur based on your skills and the skills of your partner, the skills and level of play of your opponents, and the formations utilized on each side of the net.

This simple, fun program provides tools, tactics, strategy, and simple reminders (**Ron's Riffs**) to help you as an entry-level, intermediate, or more advanced level player hit more high-percentage shots in predictable doubles play based on specific *formations* and *situations*. These simple, perhaps silly, and fun phrases help you COMMIT to the intent/purpose of your shot, position or situation and instinctively and naturally DO what you already KNOW; NOT guess or think.

As an experienced teaching pro, in my estimation, total instruction by teaching professionals is mostly delivered through private/semi-private lessons that are mostly focused on individual stroke production and mechanics for singles play compared to group lessons/clinics focused on doubles play. Learning how to properly hit/stroke the ball in general is very important, and so is where, when, and why for both singles and doubles play. However, doubles is unique because you share the court with another player, and there are two players positioned somewhere across the net.

To make it easier and more exciting for others to learn and benefit from tennis, I believe that promoting and teaching Smart Doubles® clinics and related events would be more fun and beneficial to all recreational players. *One of my favorite clinics for 3.0-4.5 players is Three and Me where I play live ball or play points and situations with and without serving to demonstrate Smart Doubles® shots, positioning, communication, and strategy.* Other effective clinic options for four or more players using a combination of drills and situational point play are Smart Doubles® Clinics #1, #2 and #3 to be discussed in more detail in Chapter 12. Welcome to Smart Doubles® School!

CHAPTER 2

THE STRATEGIC GAME OF DOUBLES

Doubles is a fun game of positioning, strategy, commitment, and communication. It requires movement up and back, left, and right depending on where the ball is and your partner's location/position. Based on your position and situation you must quickly *decide* and *commit* before you strike what you *intend* to do to the ball to execute a high-percentage shot. Otherwise, you are just swinging at a ball. In most situations you are either putting it away, putting it back in play, or unfortunately enabling your opponents an opportunity to *put it away* with a risky low- percentage shot. In doubles, the objective is to hit the best or right shot (high percentage) to the right spot or area from your current location! In other words, "play your location."

My program began and evolved while working in Atlanta from 11 years of conducting doubles strategy and positioning clinics, watching league teams and partnerships play competitive matches. Also, while in Atlanta between 1993-2004, I thoroughly enjoyed playing in the ALTA/USTA doubles leagues with and against other top players and teaching professionals. To win efficiently, is to win in straight sets or stay in control of the match. As you can imagine, it is harder to win and enjoy doubles if two singles-oriented players are sharing a court playing against the other two players who demonstrate where to be, where to place the ball, and how to communicate to make certain adjustments as the match evolves to win efficiently. As you learn and develop your strokes it is extremely helpful to apply and use them in fun games with and against similar players to help make them natural.

Upon relocating to the Bradenton/Sarasota area in 2004 and working at the #1 rated Colony Beach & Tennis Resort for four years followed by eight years at the Longboat Key Club & Resort, I began testing and using my program on resort guests, home league teams, small groups, and clinics. Given that most people who live on Longboat Key or visit this area seasonally also reside in other regions where they have taken good, bad, confusing, or misunderstood lessons and clinics. In other words, I have witnessed a lot of dumb doubles, varying opinions, philosophies, and frankly, bad advice about how people should play the game of doubles. Certain clinics are conducted for the purpose of running, exercise, competition such as cardio tennis, and variations of live ball with little to no instruction. This is a fantastic opportunity to work hard, get fit and feel like a beast. Run and gun!

Another themed option for clinics can include competitive point play or live ball with significant movement and exercise while reinforcing doubles strategy, specific tactics, formations, positioning, patience, teamwork, and finishing points. This type of clinic is ideal for partnerships, league teams and participants, and people who want to improve specifically at doubles because they play mostly doubles. This themed doubles strategy and positioning clinic can be conducted with a pro feeding to create situational live ball or serving by the participants. *The reality of doubles is sharing the court with another partner and being effective together.* They say it takes two to tango. How you move and communicate with your partner will determine your success at doubles.

Hence to offset much of what I frequently saw and heard from a wide variety of players, I began using the term *Smart Doubles*® to describe and clarify what I taught and expected to see as a coach. I saw two ways to play doubles and I wanted to reinforce the better way, the smart way in simple terms through common sense; <u>NOT</u> in terms of or related to professional-level players, their previous or current pro's playing style, preferences, or bad instruction that is just not feasible for their current skills, level, and ability.

Too often pros teach based on what they do at an advanced level or did as young players such as serve and volley. Depending on your serve, volley, and athletic skills, most recreational players will need a proper invite- short ball- to be successful at the net. My advice is to know your strengths and weaknesses and use common sense. Instead of teaching general doubles strategy and positioning clinics which sounds some-what rigid, technical, and boring, I began teaching Smart Doubles® clinics. Since I have enjoyed much success with my program as a teaching professional, I want to share it with players and other teaching professionals who work with recreational players to facilitate more success and enjoyment of doubles for this large population of players.

CHAPTER 3

THE THREE BASIC FORMATIONS

Smart Doubles® is like real estate in that both are location, location, and location-driven! Formations are your foundation for effective partnerships and success. To visually illustrate Smart Doubles®, I will provide court diagrams to create a good visual of basic formations and positions. Although there are only three possible formations on either side of the net, images 3.1 and 3.2 include examples of transition forward to the net immediately or eventually after serving or returning.

Illustrations of the basic formations: The first court diagram in image 3.1 **shows one up and one back** on both sides. This is the typical formation to begin most points in doubles. The second court diagram shows the returner's partner positioned back at the baseline creating one up and one back vs **two back**. The third court diagram shows both the SP and RP starting back at the baseline to begin the point. The fourth court diagram shows the returner moving forward after their return or eventually creating **two up** vs one up and one back. As you know, servers must serve from their baseline and the returner must allow the serve to land inside the intended box for match play.

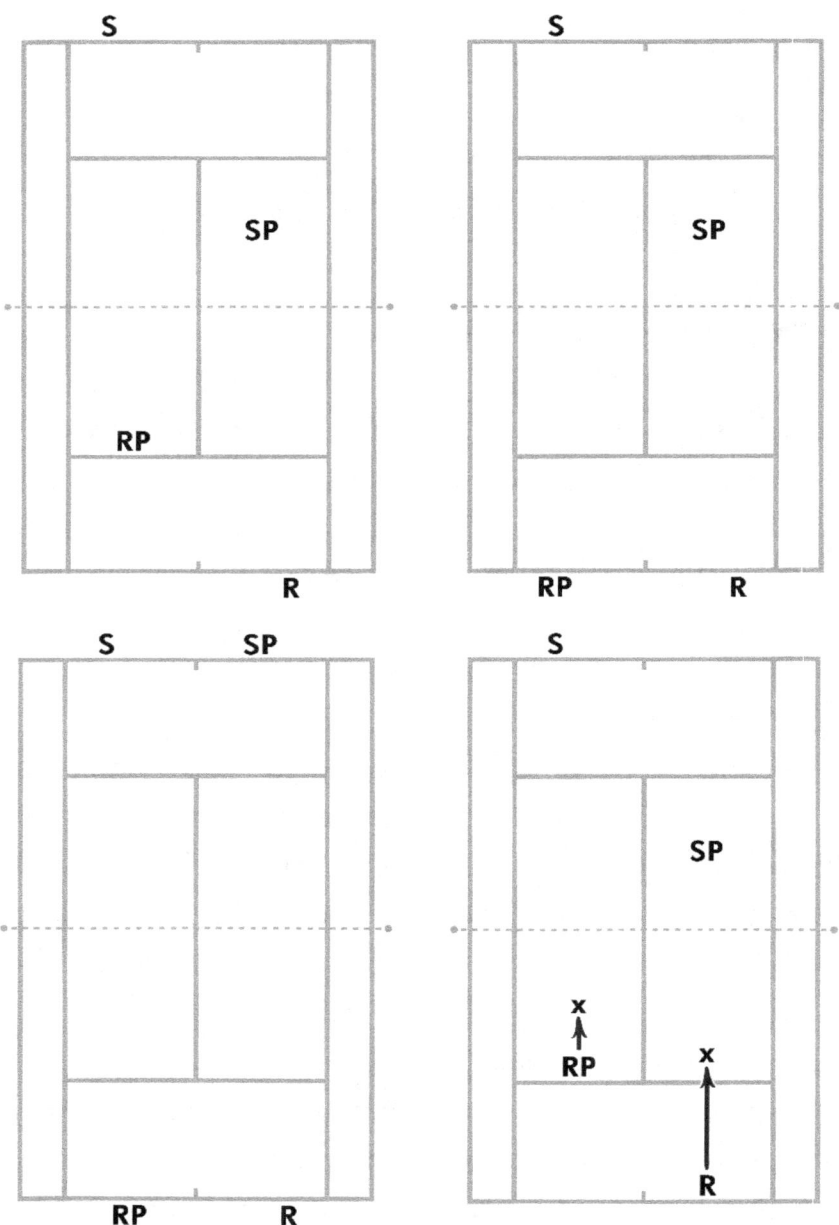

Image 3.1 shows one up, one back on both sides of the net; two back on return; two back on serve and return; and transition to two up after return.

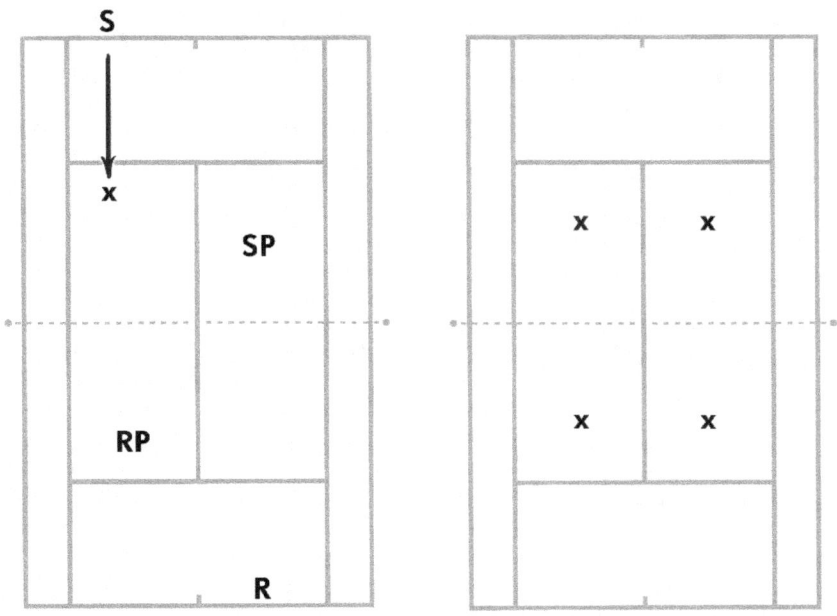

Image 3.2 shows the server moving in after their serve or eventually to create two up vs. one up and one back. Also, it shows all four players at the net for volleys.

As illustrated, there are only three basic formations from which you can play doubles on your side: one up and one back, two back and two up. The default formation is usually one up and one back on both sides of the net to start most points. This neutral formation may provide a slight strategic advantage for the up player if the deep player can keep the ball away from the opposing net player. Also, it does require that all players in these positions do their job (deep to deep, short to short, wide to wide) by playing their position/location to maximize success. Also, getting your serve in from the baseline is an especially key role, job. However, positions/formations can change quickly depending on how points and games are won or lost. Frequently asked questions are:

- When do I move forward to the net to volley?

- When do we play two back?

There are specific points, situations when playing against aggressive/stronger players, playing two back makes a lot of sense. For example, if you are playing against a strong server and your partner's return is weak and not consistently going cross court away from the opposing net player, playing two back to start makes a lot of sense. Also, if you find yourself at the net often against two up (one up and one back on your side), you are likely the target and recipient of offensive volleys and overheads to defend. Often this situation occurs when the returner comes into the net after receiving a short, weak second serve that pulls you in naturally. This short ball can also come during a cross court rally. *When you achieve two up against one up and one back you have the ideal situation/formation to finish the point quickly by forcing the opposing team to hit perfect low shots, cross court shots, down the middle shots, or a high lob.*

As you can imagine it is more challenging for one net player to defend against two net players. Based on not being able to control or be effective at the net on certain points, it is very smart to drop back with your partner to allow more time to defend, pass or lob. Also, it makes good sense to start two back at or near the baseline if your partner has a weak first or second serve and the returner is consistently targeting you at the net.

Occasionally, when you have players who prefer net play or are good at the net, you will obtain an extremely competitive formation on both sides of two up against two up. Depending on the level, usually a deep player will be invited with a short ball to approach and play at the net, or a server will approach the net after serving that creates two up. Also, returners will approach the net especially after returning weaker first or second serves. Based on who you are playing against and their strengths and tendencies, you must be aware of what formations are working and use them consistently.

As stated, real estate and doubles have something important in common: Location, location, and location! I consistently stress *"play your current location"*. In doubles there are two players on each side of the net *partnering* to beat the other two across the net. When two players are in the same offensive or defensive mode that is a good thing. It is easier for two at net to successfully take out one up at the net with middle, feet, and alley/angled shots. Two back against one up and one back makes it easier to avoid the net player in the up position and provides more time and opportunity to better control who to target, how and when. Two back is ideal when your deep partner is not playing "keep away" consistently or the opposing net player is aggressive and poaches often. Two up against two back provides more time for the back players to lob, drive down the middle, cross court, or directly target a weaker player. However, two up with good position can quickly angle the ball short off the court if the two back are not hitting perfect low or high balls. In practice-not competition- or during a warmup you can rally or volley at net directly to the deep player, but in a match, especially with good position, you want to angle or place your volleys and keep the ball away from the deep player.

My favorite formation to see my teams obtain naturally is *two up* against *one* at the net with one back. It provides the best formation and advantage from which to finish points quickly in doubles play especially if the two up are volleying (not letting the ball bounce or struggling) **Short to Short** to the middle or an alley. The transition shot to approach the net which creates the two-up formation, forces the deep player to hit a perfect lob or low pass to make the two up now at net struggle. If the deep player does not neutralize the approach, his alone partner at the net should be in big trouble dealing with a **High You Die or One and Done** volley or overhead from the opposing net players. This transition to the two up formation creates net control, pressure on your opponents, and an opportunity to finish the point quickly. Advanced level players will obtain this formation consistently seeking to win more points efficiently by controlling the net. However, in this formation, lower-level players may get lobbed or passed more often depending on the quality- angle or depth- of their approach shots and volleys.

CHAPTER 4

RON'S RIFFS

It is my pleasure to introduce my favorite part of the Smart Doubles® program which are **Ron's *Riffs***. To reinforce the foundation of Smart Doubles® during clinics, I often say ***Deep to Deep***, ***Short to Short*** and ***Wide to Wide*** to remind players to *commit* to hitting high percentage shots based on their location and situation. Of course, there are a few exceptions for specific reasons. Since the doubles game has a limited number of specific situations with three possible formations (one up and one back, two back and two up), your position/location, situation (struggling or not), and the formation of the two players across the net will determine the right shot as in the high percentage shot. To enjoy and win at doubles consistently you cannot just hit the ball and do whatever. You must conform to the unique nature and strategy of doubles, and in particular Smart Doubles® for more consistent success.

Players win or lose doubles matches for specific reasons. Both players are working together, anticipating their partner's tendencies, supporting each other, talking, and planning as they play or not. Also, people often play differently in drills, clinics and lessons compared to matches. Another example of "dumb doubles" is when one player or two are basically playing singles as in just hitting the ball across the net without a purpose or consideration of partnership. Honestly, I have seen a ton of "dumb" doubles games, and most of the time, it was not fun! For those who are new to tennis, to really enjoy doubles you must learn how to play doubles. Let's dig in!

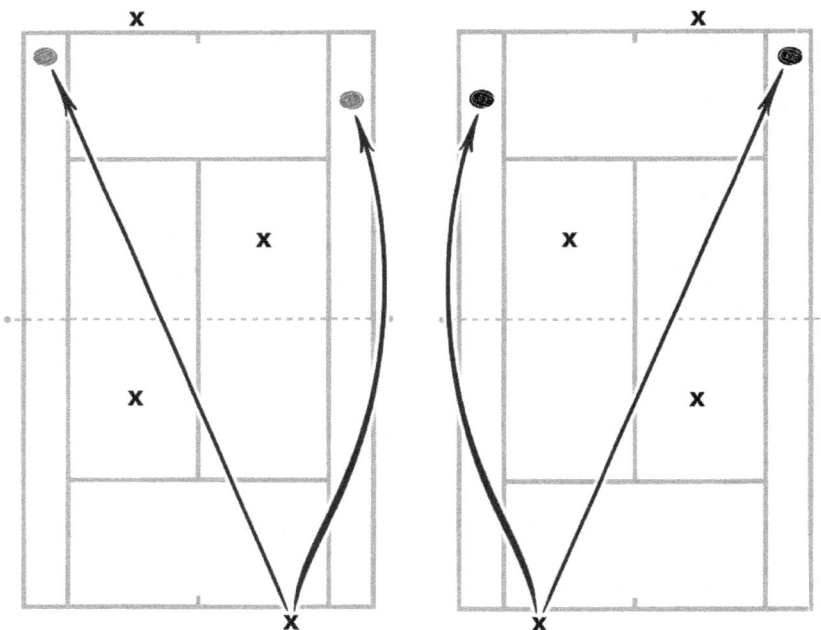

Image 4.1 is an illustration of your **Deep to Deep** options from both deuce and ad sides when your location is deep at the baseline.

Please notice your two best options! When deep at or near your baseline you should be playing keep away from the opposing net player against one up and one back across the net. Hitting deep cross court or lobbing deep are your two high percentage shots as depicted in image 4.1. This is your job and responsibility from the deep position! Again, play your location! Hitting to the alley or at the well positioned net player from, near or behind the baseline is a low percentage shot. This *deep to short example is* usually a bad idea. However, there are a couple reasonable exceptions! For example, if the net player across the net **has not moved up** *to an offensive volley position* which means their feet are exposed. Driving low at their feet or down their alley or towards their BH volley is a smart option. This low drive should make them *struggle*.

Another exception or reason to use a *deep to short* shot, especially when you are not struggling, is when the *net player is leaving too early* to anticipate your cross court shot. If they tend to be predictable or repeat offenders related to the two previous exceptions, make sure your partner is aware that you are likely to drive to their feet or alley so they can move up or drop back depending on the quality of your drive to anticipate their likely response. Otherwise, be patient and play "keep the ball away" from the net player when you are physically deep with **Deep to Deep shots.**

Often people position way too close to the net making a lob (**Deep to Deep**) an excellent option than hitting cross court. If you lob consistently in this situation, you will teach the net player a valuable lesson. Lobbing, especially from the deuce or right side that forces a switch, provides an excellent option to move in at least to the service line to anticipate a weak return from the deep player (lob retriever) to put away **Short to Short.** Yes, the lobber was in a deep position, but the lob is hopefully deep and over the net person's head, so you will have enough time to move up to the service line area to better position for offense closer to the net as illustrated in image 4.2. I love this tactic because it makes the deep player travel to the other side of the court to struggle to return a deep BH lob retrieval. Unfortunately, the opposing net player who is not chasing down the lob, should angle back to the service line or deeper to observe where their partner is to better anticipate a weak or perhaps a good, defensive lob retrieval. Based on this lob and forced switch situation, often the net player needs to drop all the way back near the baseline to have a chance to defend their partner's short or weak lob retrieval. Also, it is okay to stay back after hitting a good lob that forces a switch. If you do stay back, the point may last longer, and you may not be able to take advantage of the struggle that you created across the net. Occasionally, your lob from the deep court may be short enabling the opposing net player to hit offensively an OH forcing your net partner back even more to protect himself and the middle! If you are struggling to get to the ball, you are likely to lob short. Prior to your contact, you may emphatically say to your partner at the net *"**BUD, BUD**"* = back up dude or "**BUB, BUB**" = back up bi#$#. I learned BUB from my wife, Brenda and I made up the other one for the guys. In this situation, a simple "back, back" will work fine! However, know the rules regarding this situation to avoid a hinderance call by your opponents.

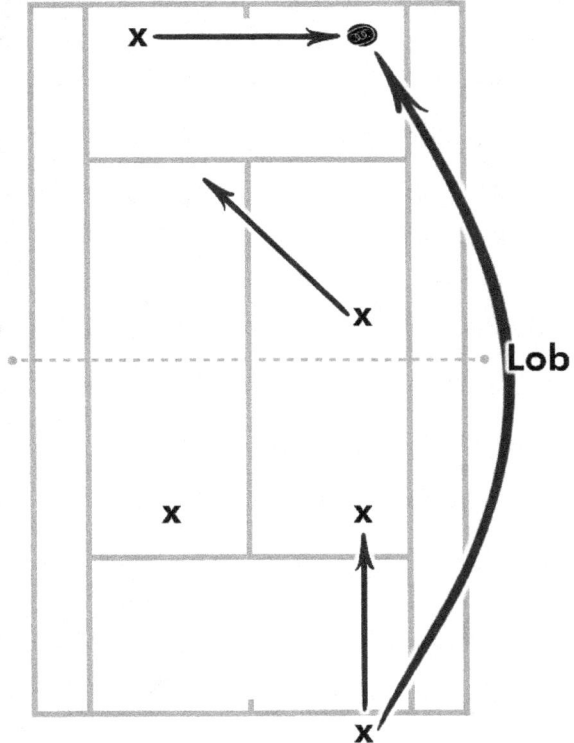

Image 4.2 shows an illustration of a deep lob, lob retrieval by the deuce court player. Lobber moves forward to zone 2-3 to finish point with OH/volley short to short. Also, it shows two up against one up retreating.

Since most doubles points are played in the one up and one back formation it is the net player's job to ***put it away*** usually to the middle or an alley as illustrated in image 4.3. As depicted, the deep player in the box can drive the ball to engage the net player or lob. The player or players at net should finish the point ***Short to Short*** if not struggling and in good position. You should not volley *short to deep* when your position is good, and your contact level is above the net. With good position volley and hit overheads ***Short to Short***! However, when your position is not good such as a low volley from the service line area or your contact level is below the net, you should try to put the ball back in play cross court away from the opposing net player and preferably deep towards the deep player. With two up against two back you may be forced to hit a few deep volleys during a point because of poor positioning and lower or tougher volleys, until a higher ball comes back that can be angled off the court.

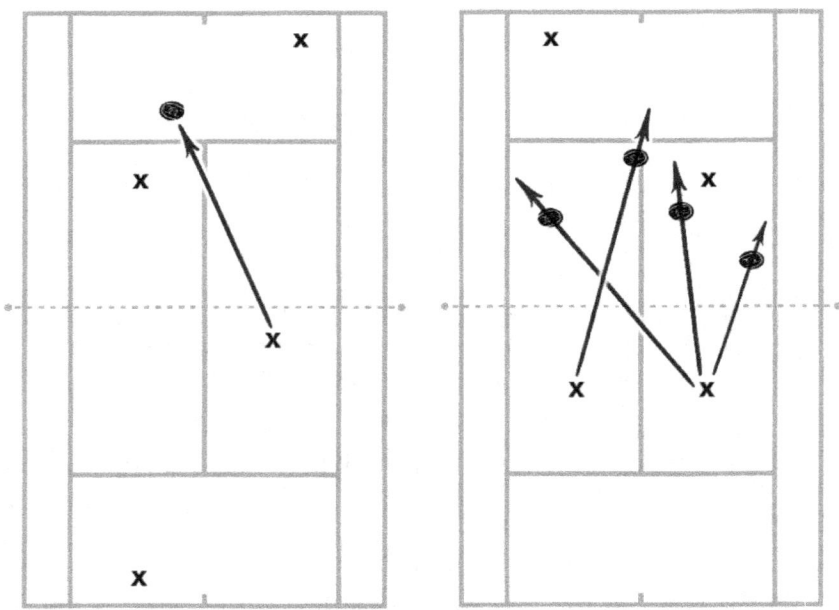

Image 4.3 shows Short to Short volleys/overheads with one up and two up against one up and one back.

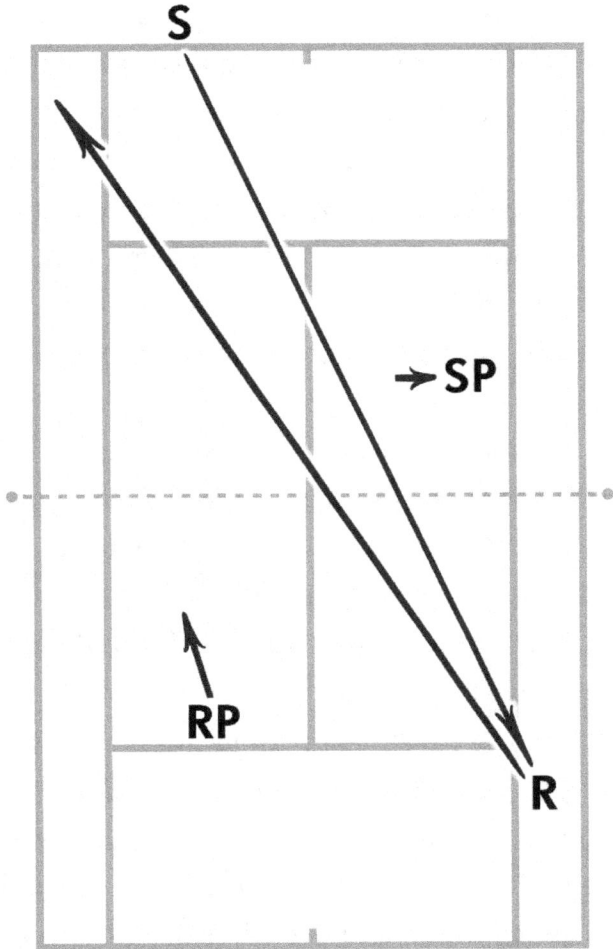

Image 4.4 shows wide to wide return against a wide serve.

When in a deep location/position and pulled wide against one up and one back you must return the ball *Wide to Wide* cross court to keep the opposing net player from volleying to your now larger middle. Image 4.4 illustrates this common situation for all players when served wide. When any player is pulled wide or off the court the space between you and your partner grows. An exception, if the opposing net player leaves his alley too early or before you strike, you may have a winning shot down the alley if you are not struggling too much. If pulled wide by the incoming deep player's approach shot or serve, a **Wide to Wide** low cross court shot at his/her incoming feet is a great option or a lob. Hitting to the middle is not high percentage when pulled wide because it leaves your middle wide open for a volley by the opposing net player. One of my students in Florida reinforces in her mind the above **Deep to Deep**, **Short to Short** and **Wide to Wide** as DSW! This acronym is easy to remember and reminds her of shopping.

Related to the deep player hitting deep cross court and staying back is the net player's job to **FTB-** *follow the ball* including on the serve which must land in the box in front of you. I encourage the server's partner at net to take a step or two left or right towards the bounce of the ball directly in front of them to better position for the likely return and potential volley. Image 4.5 illustrates the SP following the ball as in the serve, and the RP moving up for offense and towards the CC return. Too often players stand, stay too centralized or frozen in a neutral position relative to the net but not *relative to the ball after it lands* in the service box or deeper near the baseline during a cross court rally. It is hard to get involved, poach and volley more often if you are not at least slightly *following the ball*.

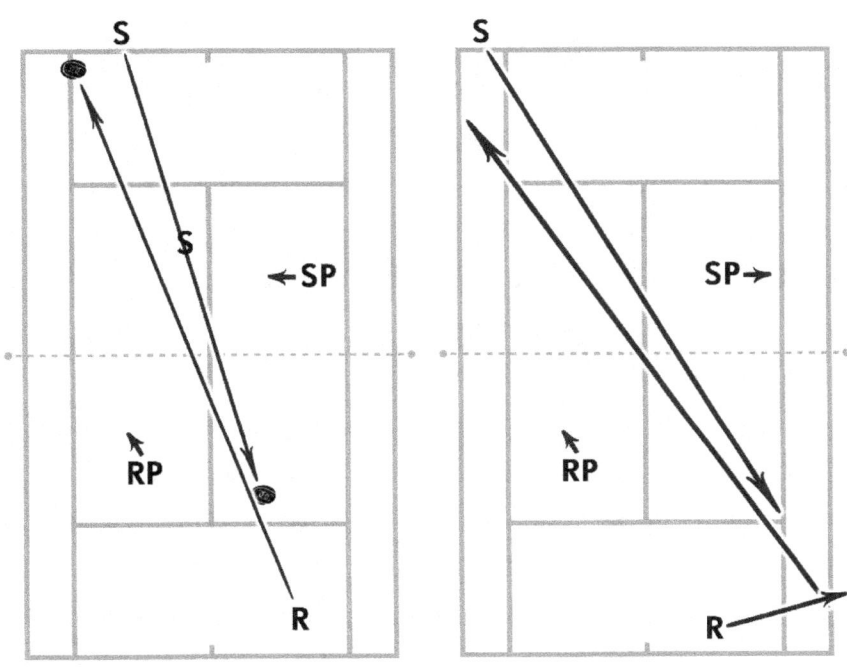

Image 4.5 shows Tennis Two Step and FTB.
Serve goes down the middle then wide on the second one.

Also, regarding movement at the net in a one up and one back format, I teach a simple dance called the *Tennis Two Step*. When the ball goes back, you take *two steps* back and wait for the ball to clear the opposing net player's racquet. Once the ball clears them at net, you move up *two steps* and towards the bounce of the ball. Before the deep player strikes in front of you, you need to be ready, balanced not on your way up. To be clear, when positioned back two steps you are in a defensive position and focused on the opposing net player; NOT your partner behind you. The opposing net player's movement in relation to the ball approaching at the net will alert you how to move next.

By watching the opposing net player, you can see where the ball is traveling as in safely clearing them or not and to move up for offense or back even more for defense. However, at times you should look back quickly after your two steps back when you know or sense your partner is pulled wide, forced up for a drop or when switching while your partner is chasing down a lob behind you. In these situations, you need to see how much your partner is struggling to quickly determine to move back to cover more court and better anticipate what is about to happen next. When your partner is struggling, he is likely to produce a weaker shot. If your partner is consistent at hitting deep and keeping you out of trouble while at net, then you are focused forward on the opposing net player, not your partner. If your partner is hitting too many balls directly to or near the opposing net player with good position, two back would be a smart formation adjustment until more balls go deep than towards the opposing net player.

Again, the mission here is to *keep it simple* and make sure you are moving back for defense and up for offense! During a normal CC rally, if you angle back two steps or more to cover more of the middle, just be sure you regain your offensive net position when the ball clears the opposing net player. Too many players just look back without moving back to position for defense. YOUR success at the net mostly depends on *your partner's deep balls, your movement and anticipation*. Also, CC angles hit by your partner in transition from zone two/NML can be a set up for put away shots. You must **FTB** to protect some of your alley based on how wide the ball goes. Often, players at the net anticipate the obvious cross court/wide to wide shot without first protecting some of their alley.

Another frequently used riff of mine is **Happy Feet**. It is imperative to maintain happy feet at the net especially in doubles play. Your movement and **Happy Feet** create a warning sign and nonverbal message that you can and will intercept more balls. In contrast, unhappy and depressed feet make it harder to reach more volleys when up in good position that can and should be yours. Also, unhappy feet make it harder to anticipate and defend attempted alley and middle shots or direct aims. If you lack confidence at the net, fake it with **Happy Feet** and movement or play back. Also, when transitioning from NML/midcourt with a cross court approach shot, I suggest making your *split step* (brief pause in forward movement) when your shot bounces across the net just before the deep player strikes. Ideally, in transition, you are seeking to obtain a good volley position inside the service box. If you pause your footwork when your ball bounces across the net you can better see, anticipate, and prepare for your next shot. If you continue moving forward after your approach bounces, you are likely to be off balance and struggle making a volley or getting back for a lob or overhead. For comparison, younger, more athletic, and advanced level players often get in good position quickly and split step at or just before the opponent makes contact. As a side note, two of my favorite and most popular Smart Doubles® retail items are Shoe Bags embroidered with **Happy Feet** and Tennis Towels also embroidered with several other riffs as key motivational reminders.

My favorite and most often verbalized riffs are related to the net player in good, offensive position. For example, when you or your partner hit high over the middle of the net or near the net player in good position that creates a **High You Die** shot opportunity for your opponent. Often this donation comes from a player in NML struggling to scoop up a low ball at their feet which creates a poaching opportunity for the net player across the net in good position. This situation is illustrated in image 4.7 on page 43. Anytime you are struggling, especially in transition or from a short location, put the ball back in play cross court, not directly to the net player in good position. In this situation you must commit to keeping the ball away from the other net guy in the *crusher, terminator, or predator* position! Also, when hitting from a deep location, trying to thread the needle down the line when the other net player is in good position is too often an easy volley opportunity especially for a better player.

Against one up and one back the ideal placement for your volley is to the middle. I call those shots **Money Middle** and **One and Done** to reinforce putting the ball away where there is no racquet. These shots are illustrated in image 4.6 on page 42. Often the ball comes back when hitting at the opposing net player's feet which are close to their racquet. At a higher level of play often the middle ball is anticipated and returned defensively. Therefore, after you **FTB** a step or two towards your awesome first volley, you may have a second shot or an easy *put away* to a left or right alley **Short to Short** to finish what *YOU* started. Hitting to the middle first between the two players *with follow- up and anticipation* of a weaker shot in return is closing out the point and sealing the deal instead of staying, watching, admiring, and allowing the struggling net player off the hook! In other words, it may take two volleys for you to finish the point.

Also, when moving to your left or right towards the center line a few steps as in poaching, usually you will naturally hit in front of your movement and balance towards the middle or the net player's feet or alley, but not behind you *short to deep* right back to the deep player. If you cross over the center line with momentum into your partner's court while hitting or attempting to hit the ball, your deep partner must automatically switch and cover your half. In other words, when moving over into the other half to strike a volley, your objective is to take out the low hanging fruit and stay. Sometimes when moving left or right towards the center line to hit a high ball when close to the net, you may be able to angle or drop the ball *short* opposite your momentum. Generally, if moving to your right, hit the middle, net player's feet, or alley in front of your movement. If moving to your left hit the middle, net player's feet, or alley in front of your movement. As discussed, hitting to the middle is ideal where there is no racquet and a more open target. However, on the move at net at times you will have to make the opposing net player struggle with your targeted volleys in his direction-low hanging fruit.

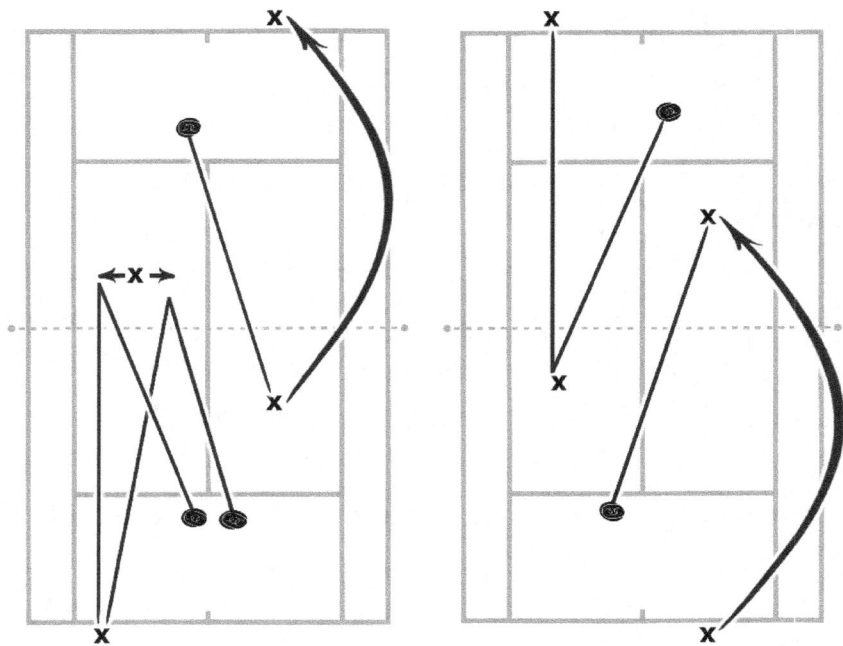

Image 4.6 shows One and Done, Money Middle and High You Die FH, BH and OH.

Opposite of **High You Die** is **Low You Go**. When you or your partner force another net player or a player in transition to hit or scoop up from below the net or from a defensive position, **FTB** a step and try to intercept an upward traveling ball since they should be struggling. This common situation is also illustrated in image 4.7.

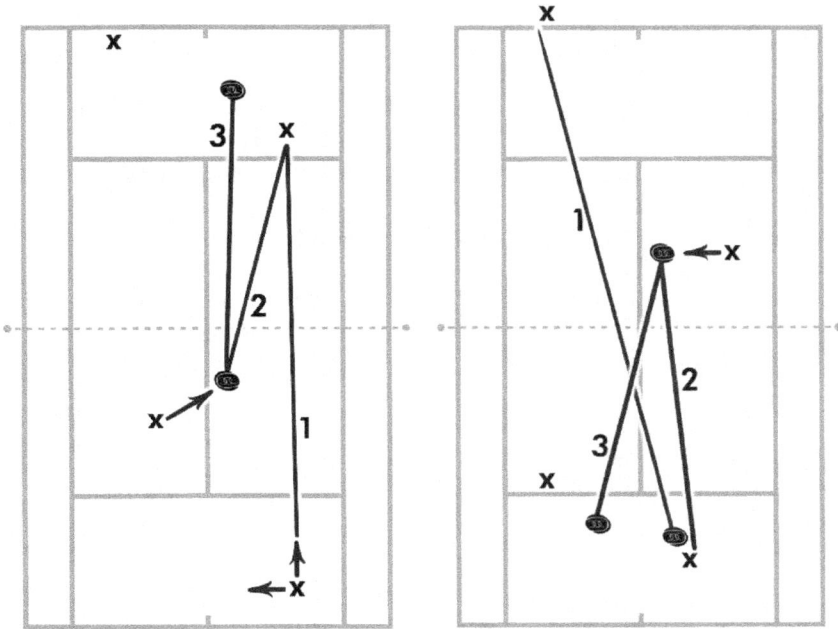

Image 4.7 shows player hitting up from NML providing a **High You Die** shot.

All my riffs are based on strategic doubles common sense. They are memorable, catchy phrases that I have heard or learned previously from other pros/players or made up or modified from my matches or from watching matches. Certainly, other teaching professionals who teach doubles strategy and positioning have their own or similar riffs that enable them to be effective as a coach. At smartdoubles.com, we are open to sharing additional riffs from our affiliates that promote and reinforce Smart Doubles®. Again, my mission is to make the strategic game of doubles easier to learn and more fun to play. In the following chapters, I will share additional riffs to reinforce more purpose, planning, intention, and commitment in your doubles play.

SMART DOUBLES

CHAPTER 5

THE IMPORTANCE OF COMMUNICATION ON AND OFF THE COURT

As stated, doubles is a game of positioning, strategy, commitment, and communication. To maximize your fun and success you must be willing to talk to your partner, share your strengths, weaknesses, and tendencies, and be aware of what it takes to put forth your best effort as a TEAM. Often communication between partners starts with, "do you prefer deuce or ad"? This question means do you prefer to return serve with your FH or BH from the left or right side of the court. While this is a great question, it is ONLY the beginning of this on-going process of talking before, during and after your match or game. In other words, the game of doubles requires effective communication and a plan that can and will change as needed based on you and your partner's skills and performance. Also, the unique skills and performance of your opponents will come into play. I love the quote from the movie, *King Richard*, that Mr. Williams used to keep especially Serena and Venice focused: "if you do not have a plan, plan to fail." [4] There is much truth in that statement that applies to sports, business, and life off the court. Also, a good plan requires a commitment to follow through with execution.

Preferably, find a partner or partners you like being around, playing with and together can make quick strategic adjustments through simple, timely communication to put forth your best effort as a team. For example, if you get lobbed while at net, please say "MINE," "I got it" or ask for help by saying quickly "SWITCH" or "YOURS." Your partner at the net should be taking and crushing short lobs. Instead of me taking away a potential overhead, that you can put away, I will wait briefly to get your reaction or commitment. So, speak up! Often, the deep player will say "switch" because the lob looks high and maybe deep, or they may see you struggling or will struggle to get back quickly to hit an offensive shot. As the net player, I suggest simple and quick communication to commit to taking it or asking for help with a switch. Saying nothing, assuming and hoping are examples of poor communication and "dumb doubles."

Another good example of the importance of communication is when the net player is moving across the center line to poach or retrieve a drop shot and moves well into their partner's half who is in a deep position. Do you stay after making your shot or go back to your side? Of course, you will stay after crossing over unless there is a good reason to cross again. This situation requires quick and decisive communication as well as having an understanding with your partner. When your partner relocates into your court during a rally, you must relocate into theirs. SWITCH!

Too often, unfortunately, players complain about their partner's inability or unwillingness to talk, plan, and strategize during a match. I understand that you may NOT always be able to execute specific shots, but it is better to know by talking what shots and positions are best against the two unique players across the net if you want to maximize your fun and success. Surprisingly, perhaps, luck will only be a small percentage of your success. As a suggestion, during play only commit to what you do well and avoid trying shots and positions/situations you lack confidence in.

Where are you serving? Can you serve to her backhand? Hopefully, your partner can commit to a target area and aim their serve. Let's play two back on this point or game for a specific reason! Shall we do the Australian on the ad or deuce point because the returner has an effective angled return or drop? What do you think? Also, being positive and encouraging helps too. Great shot, good serve, and impressive set partner! Let's not take a nap going into the second set! Let's stay focused! Good try, partner! After your partner misses a shot on a big point *try* not to show disgust or disappointment. Say, "you got the next one" or "he hit a really good shot." Maintaining positive, supportive verbal and non-verbal (body language) communication is especially important to maximize your success and fun.

Another favorite riff of mine that applies to communication between you and your partner is *What is your plan Stan*. As you play, you will see and understand what is working and what is not. Do share and discuss with your partner since it will help create more of what you want. For example, if you are playing two back, talk in advance to be sure the FH player or the better player takes the middle ball. During my clinics in

Florida, I will change this riff to **What is your plan Fran** when Fran is in my clinic, or I am coaching a lady's team. This riff reinforces that strategically, mentally, and emotionally you are aware of what it takes to perform well today and willing to do your best. Often, it comes down to simply keeping your eyes on the ball long enough to hit your desired shot; staying focused on the task at hand NOW as in planning to hit a FH cross court or letting go of the frustration from a previously missed shot. During play being worried about your abilities and thinking too much about your strokes can create too much negative *self-talk* and distractions. This inner negative chatter can interfere with your focus on the ball and your ability to effectively use your current skills. Stay positive, present, and focused on your desired outcome. Be consistent, open to growth and seek to enjoy and preferably win. Always know the score and play one point at a time! Remember, your partner is not perfect, and they will make mistakes too.

Playing with the same partner or partners as much as possible in *practice matches*, *social games* and *round robins* is ideal. Knowing your partner's strengths and weaknesses is very important too. How well do they move, anticipate, finish points, and keep the ball in play? Even taking clinics/lessons with your favorite partners is wise to be sure you are getting the same or similar coaching, so your time spent with a teaching pro enables you to be more effective together during match play. For comparison, a private lesson is about you without sharing the court with a partner or communicating with a partner about what it takes to be effective against the other two players across the net. Also, when possible, before a match schedule a 30–45-minute warmup with your partner or teammates. Going into your pre-match warmup that I refer to as a "meet and greet," *ready to play* is a great opportunity to notice what is unique about your opponents before the match begins. In other words, after meeting and greeting your opponents, now you can notice more about their unique skills (slice or topspin groundstrokes), tendencies (stands too close to net or in NML, over hits FH), apparent weakness, strengths, mobility issues, serve placement and pace or avoidance of certain shots such as overheads or backhands. Paying some attention to your opponents' tendencies during your very brief warmup will help both of you focus and commit to *specific shots and formations,* and a *plan* especially when in the deep court, serving and returning. For example, share with your partner that one player is left-handed, but seems not to be the better player. The other player seems to over hit and is inconsistent. Agree to hit more balls to this player when they are deep and maybe at net to take advantage of the weaker player. Help them hit more unforced errors and forced errors. Perhaps one player stands too close to the net, one player has a weak backhand groundstroke or BH volley, and the other player cannot move quickly. Based on what you have observed and will see during the match keep three or more balls in play, lob, find their BH, angle or drop. In competitive play, if you fail to notice and share such tendencies about your opponents, you will enable them to play well and likely beat you easily until you eventually make a few key discoveries. *Certain tendencies about your opponents are more obvious to notice if you are already warmed up and ready to play.* Once the match begins, opportunities to talk, adjust and plan are between points, games, and sets.

When I am not serving, I walk back to my server with a ball in hand to suggest something that will help me be more effective at the net and help my partner hold serve. Often, in between points, we confirm our strategy and support each other. For example, can you serve at their body or backhand? Serve to their backhand and I will poach as he hits. This returner has a great lob that we have struggled with, so I will stay back on this point. Signals are helpful but they need to be discussed and practiced with your partner. In addition, you can always find a better way to say something "us" or "we" oriented that is short and simple that encourages your partner. For example, let's keep the ball in play cross court longer when the weaker player is serving and returning. Remember you are a team, and no one likes to be told during a match/game what they are doing wrong. If you play mixed doubles with your spouse or significant other, your encouragement or lack of will go all the way home. What you say and how you say it matters. More things to practice-Argh!

CHAPTER 6

MORE ON FORMATIONS AND
TRANSITION TO THE PARTY

S mart doubles entails being patient from the deep area of the court keeping the ball in play or deep and waiting for a shorter ball in zone two/NML that feels like an invitation to attend the party to maximize your success at net. As depicted in image 6.1, the area between 2-D and 2-C is known as No Man's Land. When your feet allow you to hit a ball between 2-D and 2-C, you should be able to follow that shot forward and position inside the service line for offensive play. My verbal riffs when the ball is short are *It's Party Time, Go to the Party* or you have been *Invited to the Party*. This means that your feet and the ball you are striking are short enough inside your baseline to attack the other deep player and force your opponent to beat you with a perfect pass or lob. Often, the ball lands so short that it forces you to come in but in a defensive manner. Since you are likely hitting up, keeping the ball away from a net player may be difficult. Some short balls are comfortable and easy to get to with more control and others will be more challenging. Either way it is an approach shot since you are moving forward towards the net.

While working at the Colony Beach & Tennis Resort on Longboat Key, we offered several scheduled daily clinics and often hosted groups and teams from all over the world. Often, during these 4-6 person clinics, I conducted a combination of feeding and point play drills that involved transition to the net for net play with two up. To motivate these players and properly teach them when and how to approach the net, I sold my transition drills, games and exercises as *invites to the party*. NO invite, NO party, stay home and keep the ball in play! Often from the baseline with two players back, one uninvited player would try to go solo without his partner to the party seeking instant gratification at the net. Also, I conducted transition and point play drills with one up and one back on both sides of the net giving an invite-shorter ball- to the deep player to transition to the net. The shorter feed that is comfortable to get to and do something with intentionally, is the *Party Ball*! It is the ball or feed that provides good options to set you up for success by attacking either player. Since all our guests were staying at the resort to have loads of fun, my party lingo worked and stayed in my teaching vocabulary to help my students transition to the net properly and play smart while at net.

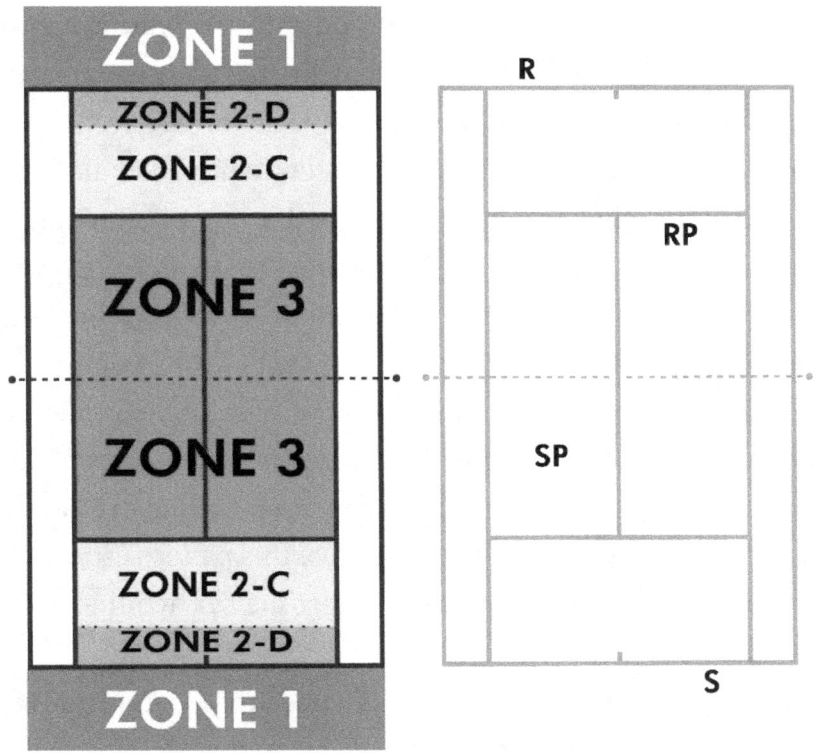

Image 6.1 shows deep, transition and put away zones and the standard one up and one back formation to start most points.

The court diagram on the right in image 6.1 shows how most doubles points begin. The server and returner are deep, the SP is positioned in the *Put Away* zone, and the RP is at or just inside the service line. The SP has the advantage because the serve must land in the box directly in front of them. The RP cannot move forward until the return clears the opposing net player and goes cross court. The net players are moving up and back during the rally- *Tennis Two Step*- and the deep players are being patient hitting deep to deep shots. The left court diagram is an illustration of court zones to illustrate when to attack and go to the party and when to stay at home. Often, deep players ask me "when should I go to the net"? My response is always "when you are invited"! We all have different skills, shot making abilities and levels of athleticism. Zone 2-D stands for "too deep" for most recreational players to approach the net, so put the ball back in play CC or lob as in *Deep to Deep*. Zone-1, Deep Zone ranges from behind the baseline to a step or two just inside your baseline. Hitting and moving forward from these deeper zones should frequently force you to hit low, struggling volleys from behind or near the service line. You do not want to continue this pattern especially if you cannot consistently get to at least the service line to hit good volleys.

Zone 2-C stands for "come in" because your improved hitting location *on your side* will give you a better chance of moving forward to obtain a good volley position inside the service line. Zone 2-C begins when your feet are three to four steps inside the baseline near the dotted line to indicate the NML area. As discussed in the return chapter, when the ball comes back short and *without struggle,* you have three excellent options to attack the net player (drive to their alley or middle or lob), and two options to attack the deep player (drop or drive angle) depending on how short you are in the court. In other words, you can move forward to volley and hit overheads with more success when you are *invited* and hitting from or near Zone 2-C better known as NML. Instead of hitting CC and approaching the net, you should mix it up by attacking the net player with shorter balls-no struggle- especially if the deeper player is the better player. No one hits deep all the time and shorter balls will come during cross court rallies and from second serves. How they come- comfortable or difficult- and where your feet are when hitting shorter balls will help you to quickly determine your best option of how to transition forward to volley or attack the net player.

Additionally, you will often be forced up to the party towards the service line to retrieve a short, low ball that lands in Zone 2-C or even shorter. If struggling to get there just put the ball back in play CC deep to give you time to get in good position at the net. This is a safe, smart shot. Faster and more advanced players may be able to finesse a drop or angle wide when forced up. However, you or your partner may get lobbed when forced up. When forced up to the party, your partner if at net should move back at least slightly to cover a potential lob. This will create a staggered formation in anticipation of a lob. When your approach shot goes short to deep you are certainly enabling a likely lob. When not struggling especially, I prefer to see my students get low to hit a *Sweet Roll* as in an angled shot- usually with topspin but "slice is nice" too- placed short towards the wide alley than towards the narrow baseline. This is an excellent example of a *Short to Short* that creates more struggle for the deep player thus making the lob and passing shot a bit more challenging.

Crashing the net/party requires more skill, better footwork, and athleticism such as serve and volley and return and volley. More advanced players with better serves and returns tend to implement this direct attacking strategy to apply pressure. If the ball is bouncing at your feet consistently when positioned at or behind the service line in transition to the net, you are either moving slowly or not committed to going to the party as you strike or you are coming in from a deeper location for your skills. One of the toughest shots in doubles is an in-transition low cross court volley that goes perfectly deep to the baseline to the deep player. The more you are in the position to attempt this tough volley especially from behind or at the service line the more you should see the opposing net player poaching with a *Low You Go*. Also, if you do manage to hit your CC volley away from the eager net lady, the deep partner has three good options to beat you depending on the quality of your volley. One is to lob, the other is a low passing shot to one of the alleys, and the third is to drive down the middle. The quality of his lob or pass attempt depends on where and how the volley lands. Certainly, a CC lob has more area to land and is an excellent option. Now with both up at the party, you will need to anticipate well in this situation based on the bounce of the ball the deep player is hitting (low, high, deep, wide) and the racquet face before or at contact. Also, you need to notice the deep player's situation as in struggle or not and timing to better anticipate their likely lob or drive.

WHY come in especially when uninvited to likely struggle with a low ball at your feet in NML? The main purpose for approaching the net is to win the point quickly with two well-positioned attack racquets with anticipating *Happy Feet* inside the service box. With an angled approach shot or drop shot both players now at net should be in good position and ready to put away the ball *Short to Short* with an overhead or volley. This angled approach opens the court for a well-placed put away shot to the middle or alley. Again, the frustrating and effective lob comes into play when you enable the lob with a slower or medium pace cross court approach shot hit from either a short or deep location directly back to the deep player's racquet. When your partner's approach shot practically enables an easy or likely lob, you must proactively move back some-stagger-to anticipate the lob.

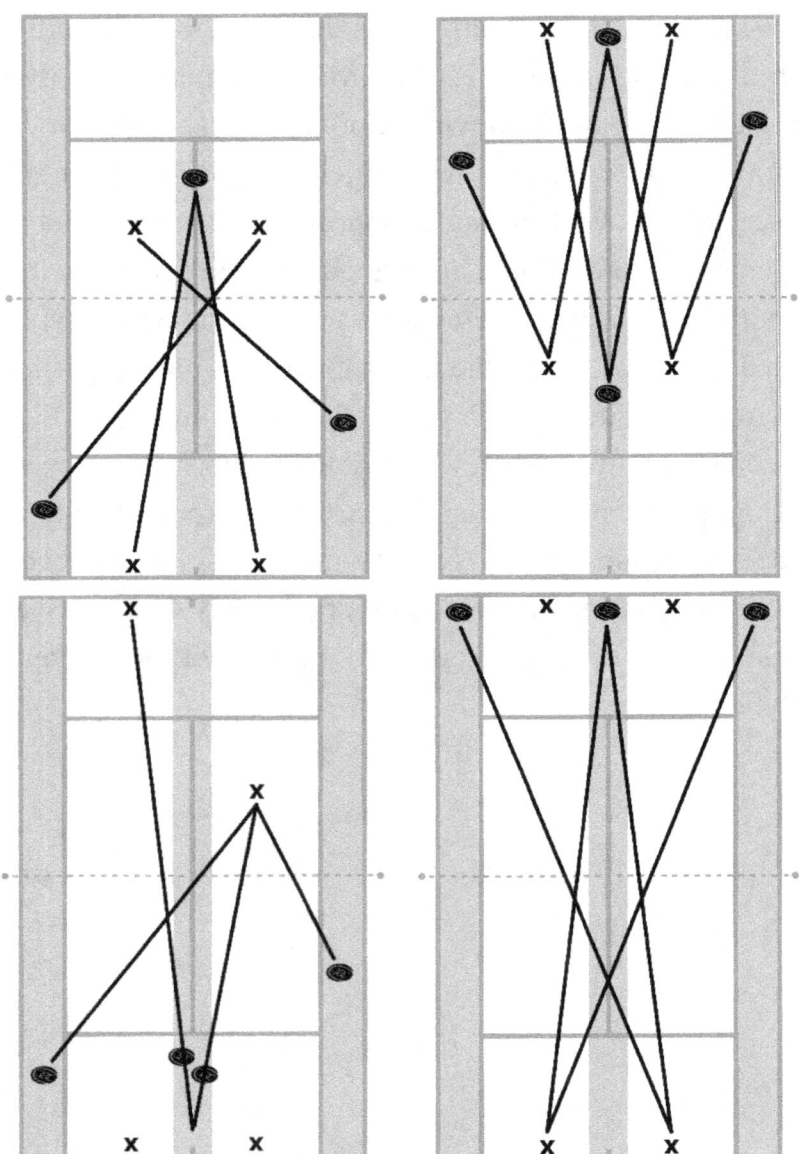

Image 6.2 shows court diagrams of the three alleys with various formations: Top two courts show high percentage groundstroke and volley/OH shot options for two up vs two back. The bottom two courts show high percentage groundstroke and volley/OH options for one up vs two back, and high percentage groundstroke shots for two back on both sides of the net.

Image 6.2 is a modified illustration of the three alleys that I first saw in Sherry Bedingfield's book *A Tennis Guide for Women*.[2] I have not had the opportunity to work with Sherry, but I know she was a great collegiate coach in Tampa, Florida. Most people think of the court with two alleys than three. There is a popular riff "***down the middle solves the riddle***" that pertains to offensive shots hit from the net with great position down the middle, and from the baseline in certain situations. These diagrams show three alleys instead of two and provide a great visual to help you mentally commit to the purpose, placement and intent of your shots when playing. Knowing your location on the court and the formation across the net helps you to commit your eyes on the ball instead of looking up at your desired target. As you can see from the top two court diagrams in image 6.2, the two up with great position have a brief moment to finish the point against two back with angled volleys and overheads. They are now seeking instant gratification from winning the point quickly. If they volley or hit deep even to the middle, they risk getting lobbed. But hitting to the middle is better than hitting directly back to their racquets. With two up against two back it is a good idea to only volley deep when the ball is low or when your position is not great as in struggling with a deep lob. The back players against the two up players have more time and a terrific opportunity to hit high percentage groundstrokes to the middle initially to create struggle followed by a lob, cross court alley shot or down one of the traditional doubles alleys.

The bottom two diagrams show two back against one up and one back, and two back against two back. In the one up against the two back it is important for the up player to FTB and hit well placed volleys to finish the point. Also, the back player can either target the weaker player or hit down the middle to create confusion. The last court diagram on the bottom shows how to play smart when all players are back hitting groundstrokes. This is a smart formation when players are not very comfortable at the net. Hitting to the middle alley initially followed by the cross-court alley or down the line to the doubles alley, should eventually create struggle such as a shorter ball to attack or forced errors from your opponents at the baseline. When two players are invited up together you have a unique advantage if you are not consistently enabling the lob. Also, when two players are playing back, you can target the middle alley or target a weaker player.

As mentioned previously, your best formation from which to win efficiently is two up against one up and one back. You can serve or return and transition to the net or you can be patient and wait for the *party ball* or a deep lob to transition forward. With all shorter balls that land in the NML region you want to maximize your chance of success not minimize it. Please note you receive the invite, and you give the invite as well. Eventually, during your **Deep to Deep** rallies the ball will land relatively short, and your feet will enable you to move forward to get inside the service line for quality shots. Decide and commit quickly depending on where you are hitting from-deeper or shorter location. For example, the ball and situation may be comfortable for attacking with options or low to put back in play cross court or too deep and stay back. It is okay to stay home if you do not feel invited, pulled in or forced to go to the party! For many recreational players when serving from the baseline or returning better serves does not mean you must move forward to the net to attempt to volley. You can always move back to the baseline area and rally cross court or **Deep to Deep** to play doubles. Going to the party after your deep lob is an excellent transition opportunity.

Your ability to transition to the net for success against the deep player is determined by *your hitting location,* the *type of ball* you have to hit, and where you hit it- short, angle or deep. Your ability to attack the net player is determined by *your hitting location,* the *type of ball* you have to hit, and how you hit it- low, aggressive. Either you are comfortable getting to a shorter ball or you are struggling. Quickly determine your opportunity to attack the net player or transition with a CC approach shot to hopefully be successful at net. Lastly, attacking the net player to their alley or middle with shorter landing balls is just a bonus if the server has a weak serve or the deep player is not able to hit **Deep to Deep**.

SMART DOUBLES

CHAPTER 7

SERVE, RETURN AND
TRANSITION TO THE PARTY

As you know, the game of doubles begins with either a serve or return, and the serve must land inside the service box to start a real game. In chapter 9, I will discuss in more detail alternative ways to play and enjoy doubles without a traditional serve. Smart Doubles® is about serving such that your partner has a good chance to volley at the net. Serving wide to the righty's forehand from the deuce is great approximately 25% to 35% of the time unless there is good reason to do more, such as, serving to a lefty's weaker backhand on the deuce side. This wide serve and smaller target will move your partner at net slightly wide towards the alley to cover a small area of the court. With too many wide serves and right-handed forehand returns cross court could mean the server is hitting all the balls while your partner at net is watching more tennis than participating. Placing the serve 70-80% up the middle at the body or to the right-handed returner's backhand on the deuce side is ideal. This serve placement allows your partner to move closer to the likely return trajectory of the ball at net to potentially intercept more attempted cross court returns with a FH volley. In addition, for a righty returner, the backhand cross court (inside out) from the deuce court is a more challenging return to keep away from the net player. Often a righty returner on the deuce side will position slightly to the left to hit more forehands to start the point.

On the ad side, a lefty will often struggle hitting their backhand cross court (inside out) away from the opposing net player. A lefty will likely prefer to return from the ad side to hit more strategic FH options. If returning or serving on the deuce side a lefty will often position to the right to hit more strategic FH options. Therefore, knowing and discussing serve placement in between points and games with your partner helps the server's partner to anticipate getting involved for more **One and Done** volleys and perhaps overheads while in great position at net. This planning and involvement will help the server hold serve. A brief discussion promotes a unified plan, strategy, anticipation, and good partnership-Smart Doubles®. To help implement your serve placement and your partner's intentions (stay, fake, poach) after your serve lands, you can use certain signals or verbalize them quietly to your partner with "French Toast" for serving to the FH or "Bed and Breakfast" for body-backhand or "Bacon for Breakfast." Personally, I do not eat bacon, but I love serving it up in doubles! Obviously, your plan will fail occasionally, but at least you have one. Lastly, regarding signals, using the middle finger to indicate serve placement or movement is not recommended.

Ideally, the server tries to make the returner guess and struggle with various placement patterns, speed, and spin. Just "getting it in" can make it harder to hold serve consistently in competitive matches. If you are struggling placing your serve, try first committing, both visually- looking- and mentally- imagining- what you intend for placement and type of serve before you toss, and do not chase bad ball tosses relative to your target. *LIG* means **"let it go"** regarding bad ball tosses. After tossing only hit the ones you like and know will help you hit your desired target area. As a side note- *LIG* can also apply to inflammatory situations on and off the court! My best advice regarding your serve is to take some lessons or clinics (stroke clinic-3-6 participants) that will include working on the serve to be sure your basic mechanics, motion, awareness, and patience are moving in the right direction. Secondly, practice your serve on your own for a few minutes on a regular basis and make it fun. Your best investment in your tennis game is practicing your serve on your own to reinforce a good toss, contact, feel, balance, patience, and keeping your eyes up on the ball. Aiming for a large target such as the middle of the box is a good idea to help get more serves in. Keep in mind the ball goes where you direct it, not where you hope and wish. Preferably, aim and feel as if you were simply throwing a ball with your serving arm and stay in control. In fact, to help learn the basic motion of serving at a young age or early stage of development, I highly recommend establishing first in muscle memory the kinetic chain of the throwing motion with a tennis ball, baseball, or smaller football to create the foundation for a better serve. The **serve** is a whole-body motion from your legs up to your hitting hand, and every part has to flow into the next part to achieve smooth execution.

More advanced players hit harder and deeper serves-landing on or closer to the service line- with more pace, top or slice spin that make them more challenging to return. This bigger type of serve may force the returner to move back a few steps into a defensive mode. The smart return if you can get your racquet strings on the ball is a cross court return or lob away from the net player if possible. After your defensive return, you should return quickly to your baseline area to prepare to rally ***Deep to Deep***. Usually, against better servers you are not invited to the net after returning. Also, your partner may drop back when you are struggling to return bigger serves or a certain type of serve. Consequently, if you are struggling with your return the opposing net player has an advantage and easy opportunity to end the point with a ***Short to Short*** shot that can include attacking your partner directly, if at net. Many players have a big first serve when they get it in, but the second serve is much softer and predictably easier for the returner to be more aggressive or strategic with their return. The opposite of the bigger serve is the shorter, weaker, and predictable serve with less pace and spin that either sits up high or stays low after bouncing. This shorter and weaker serve provides a consistent opportunity to transition to the net with an official ***Invite To The Party!*** Technically, the serve is a short ball because it must land in the service box. But not all serves are attackable.

Most recreational players will have a predictable pattern with how and where they serve. Therefore, based on receiving a first or second serve at least plan instead of allowing the server to totally control the point and game. Your movement up, back, left, or right *overtly* prior to the serve or toss can throw off the server and force the server out of a good rhythm. Especially, on a typical second serve, I suggest you move slightly left or right (**Operation Second Serve**) and move in a step or two to obtain a FH or BH to hit a planned shot with purpose and intent. Your modified return position and movement up, left, or right prior to the serve can throw off the server and force a double fault on occasion. Bingo! In competitive matches when the server is consistently missing their first serve, **Operation Second Serve** can provide a big advantage by allowing you to obtain the return you want against a safe or typical second serve.

When returning a weaker serve you should commit to one of two specific cross court transition options to make the server struggle and win the point with two up at net. One is a drop, and the other is an angle- **Sweet Roll**. Your drops do NOT have to be perfect or pretty with lots of underspin. They just need to be preferably lower over the net and short inside the service box that will force the server to run up and struggle. In transition to hit a shorter angled return **Get Low to Hit Low**. To mix it up you can put the ball back in play cross court and move back depending on your returning location.

Three additional options for attacking weaker serves are to drive low to the alley or middle towards the net player or lob the net player. After you make your shot towards or over the net player, wait slightly to be sure you see struggle before moving forward to the net to finish the point. If your alley shot is low or at their feet, the ball and their racquet are below the net, and she is hitting up. Good for you, and *Low You Go*! Also, if your lob is effective over their head, you have an excellent opportunity to move forward to obtain a better position at the service line area to finish the point quickly with an angled or middle shot or a power shot towards the retreating net guy.

If you are holding serve consistently, great. However, you must figure out how to break serve more often. Your best opportunity to break is when returning weaker or second serves. That is why I use in my Smart Doubles® program ***Operation Second Serve*** and ***What is Your plan Stan*** to make it easier to utilize these five specific options against second or weak serves depending on the situation. However, if the server's partner drops or plays back on either the first or second serve, you have additional options such as returning the ball directly to the weaker player or down the middle or dropping the ball short depending on how short the serve lands in the box. In the game of doubles things can change and some things stay the same such as a weak server. Therefore, you must communicate with your partner, be open to mixing it up and making adjustments throughout the match.

Other than hitting the ball out, the worst thing you can do especially when inside NML or near the service line is to return a weak/short serve (no struggle) deep and right back to the server's racquet and rush in or sit there in NML. You may get away with this shot occasionally against lower-level players. This *short to deep* return shot is likely to enable a lob or an offensive shot in return unless you hit perfectly on the baseline. The baseline is narrow and near the server's racquet, and the alley is 4.5 ft wide. *Second service returns in some fashion should make the server struggle or the server's partner struggle.* In other words, the more you plan and attempt to execute specific returns, especially on second serves, the more you will break serve! The more you break serve the easier it is to win matches given you are holding your serve most of the time. I have seen and heard much success from many of my students in response to me repeatedly saying "do something with it" related to short, fluffy weak second serves. Many of my students from my regular Three and Me clinics have shared with me how they have consistently benefited from my coaching about being aggressive and deliberate with **Operation Second Serve**. Returning a typical second serve is an opportunity to do something strategic and on purpose so take advantage!

Image 7.1 illustrates five *planned in advanced* return options as **Operation Second Serve** to attack weaker second serves being hit from inside the baseline: Short low drive down the middle or doubles alley to engage a weaker BH volley; angled approach shot to move the server wide; drop shot to make server struggle; or lob. When the serve is slower and higher the lob is an excellent option. For a righty on the ad side, moving to the left to hit a FH down the middle over the lower part of the net is an excellent option compared to a backhand hit down the doubles alley. Also, a righty on the deuce side can easily target the doubles alley with a low FH drive. A lefty returner has all the same specific options to target the SP with a low drive or the server with an angled drive or drop. All attacking returns are intended short or angled except the lob to create more struggle. In other words, plan before the serve what you intend to do.

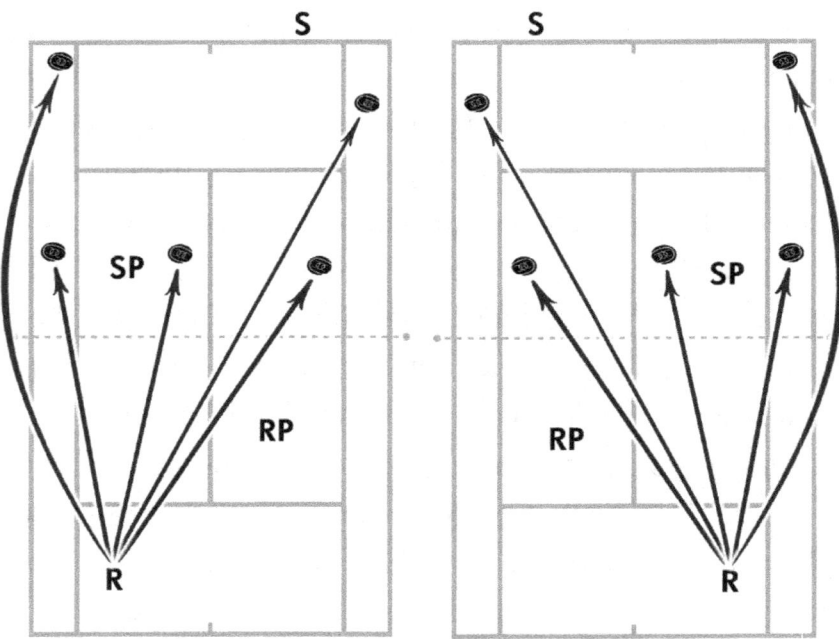

Image 7.1 shows return options for attacking second serves: lob, drive to alley or middle, drop or angle.

As stated, there are two ways to go to the party. One is to be invited and the other is to crash the party. "Crashing the party" means you are returning cross court from a deeper location or serving from the baseline (Zone 1) and moving in towards the service line in hopes to volley. Depending on the speed and placement of the serve, the speed and angle of the return, and the party crasher's footspeed, the server or returner may or may not get to or inside the service line to hit an offensive volley. Remember, the purpose for going to the party is to finish the point quickly with a forced error from struggle or a put away volley or OH *Short to Short*. Often, I say, "take the low hanging fruit" as in target at, behind or in front of the closest net player when you get well inside the service line.

This serve and move into the service line area playing style and tactic will certainly apply more pressure on the returner to hit a perfect low cross court shot or lob. Returning low at the server's incoming feet is a smart shot making the server hit up with a low volley. As you can imagine, more skill and athleticism are required to place the serve and defend such shots effectively and consistently. At times you and your partner will serve or return and position well inside the service line effectively to win many points with an attacking, well placed volley or overhead. Recently, one of my Sarasota students who usually hits a firm FH return was playing at sectionals at the USTA campus in Orlando. Once the server started serving more to her BH on the deuce side, she was able to move slightly left to use the cross court *Sweet Roll* we worked on previously with less pace, more spin and angle to make the server hit up and struggle while keeping the opposing net player from poaching.

My advice is do not "crash the party" unless you can defensively volley or half volley low from your feet around the service line or drop back quickly to cover a lob over your partner's head. Also, you should practice and improve upon this tactic, but preferably when you can afford to lose the point or are desperate to try something different to mix it up. With **Operation Second Serve** your angled return, drop and lob are all *invites to the party* to make the server struggle and make it harder for the server to beat you now with two up at net. It is certainly a great feeling and fun to win transitioning towards the net.

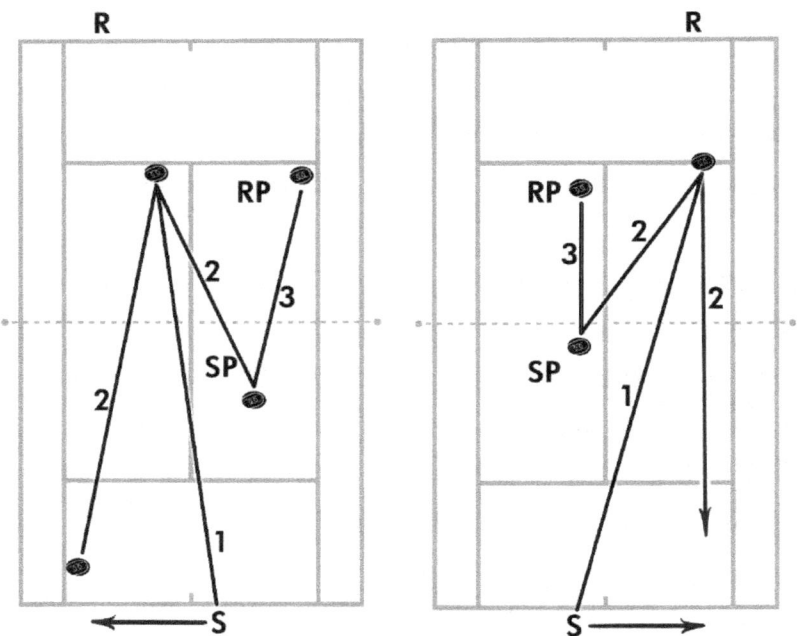

Image 7.2 shows Australian formation for lefty and righty servers.

Another variation of one up and one back is serving in the Australian formation. It is an excellent tool/tactic when you are having trouble winning especially the ad court point for certain reasons. Often during a game, the score goes back and forth from deuce to ad too many times. For current competitive players as you know this is frustrating. Usually, the ad court returner is or should be the better, tougher, the more consistent player or returner who likely prefers their backhand return from the ad side. This ad court player may be noticeably the stronger player with more consistency or weapons such as drops, angles, approach shots and net play. Perhaps the righty server has a weaker serve or backhand and cannot play consistently or effectively against the opposing ad court deep player and returner.

One simple adjustment is to use the Australian formation. BUT you must be willing to use it especially when you NEED it and NOT just know about it. Notice in image 7.2 after serving the server moves over towards the alley and the server's partner stays! The Australian formation is a game changer and puts pressure on the ad player to change their return immediately under pressure. The best application is when the score is 0- 40, 30- 40 or 40-30, or ad in or out. By talking in between points, either the server or SP can suggest this tactic. The purpose of this basic application is to simply get the serve placed to the BH to force the return out or DTL away from the net player since this is not their normal return pattern. Sometimes the return will come back up the middle, which is a good opportunity for the well positioned, not moving net player. Depending on the server's skill and placement you can use the Australian on the first serve only or on both. However, if the returner on the ad side is favoring a strong, inside- out FH, this formation may or may not work especially on a second serve. The surprise alone of using the Australian with a forced change of return especially under pressure is a game changer. For 3.0-4.5 players, keep it simple and use it especially on big points!

Another more advanced option is to serve towards the T on the ad side to a righty's FH, but the server's partner needs to be able to move towards the likely return to volley. The purpose of this serve placement and application is to get the SP more involved. In the Australian formation, if the serve is placed to the BH or body, often the return goes out under pressure because the returner should try to hit down the line away from the net player or lob. Returning directly to the net player who is now blocking their regular cross court return is a low percentage shot especially against a good serve. Holding your position at net in the Australian is important to force the returner to do something different. Ideally, you want the return to go out or directly to or near the net player for a put away shot by holding your position. If the returner escapes the pressure, the righty server moves over to hit a FH as their second ball. For a server with a weaker BH using this tactic is smart and proactive. Eventually, if used consistently, the returner will lob deep or maybe short. But the pressure is on the returner to change if used.

In addition, if a lefty is serving at 0-30, 15-40 or 40-40, using the Australian on the deuce side makes sense with the lefty aiming up the middle or T to a righty's BH or body. If the return goes deep or short down the line/alley back to the server, the lefty server will rally with her FH deep to deep until an opportunity to attack a short ball. Initially, I encourage the SP to *stay* most of the time (fake occasionally) like a puppy and wait for a treat unless there is a lob or short ball while the server moves over after serving. The basic objective is to make the returner lose the point quickly with an attempted down the alley return, and to take away their effective cross court action.

Recently, one of my newer 3.5 Longboat Key students shared with me that she and her partner used the Australian successfully on the ad side against a very good service return drop shot. The day before this friendly, fun match, we worked on it on the ad side to offset a server's weaker backhand. In a text message, she said it worked like a charm! In recreational match play, I see many good opportunities to use the Australian formation especially on big points. In other words, just do it and do not make it complicated. Again, the basic objective is to make the returner hit down the line or change directions to either help you get you back into the game or close it out with a little added pressure. The more advanced option is to serve towards either T on the deuce or ad side to get the SP involved in tracking down the anticipated return. How many more deuce, ads will you play and how long are you willing to play one service game? As a coach, it is frustrating to teach and explain this simple tactical formation in clinics to help end service games, but not see it used in matches. It does work with a little practice especially at 40-30, 30-40 or 0-40 to turn things around quickly. I am excited when I see or hear that it worked because of using it. Recently, two of my 3.5-4.0 Longboat Key students used the Australian formation during a tie breaker in a third set serving at 9-10 to the ad side. This particular returner had a good BH slice that made it harder to win ad court points. The server's partner suggested using the Australian and to place her serve up the middle towards her FH to take away her low angled BH CC return. Good idea! The return was hit into the net while the server moved to her right to anticipate a FH return towards her alley. That single point turned that tie breaker around and they won the set and the match. Clap, clap! I love hearing how my students won their matches! From 3.0 and above the simple to more advanced application of the Australian formation can be a game changer. Do not wait to use it until you are losing and desperate.

The last variation of the one up and one back related to serving and returning is the I formation or some modified version of the I formation. Depending on your ability to get up and move quickly to the left or right after the serve has landed and your partner's ability to serve over you, I reserve this tactic for advanced levels, juniors, and professionals. However, with the Australian, you can stay, fake, and move based on your skills as needed to be effective on big points. Also, the SP at net is not in the path of the serve since both are on the same half of the court initially, and the serve is going away from them at net. There is no need to dip or crouch down in fear of being hit with the serve. This formation can be very disruptive when used, but you must use it early when struggling to win certain points especially on the ad side. Success comes from practicing and using these formations with a partner who is open to winning important points, important games, and tough matches.

SMART DOUBLES

SEEING THE BALL BETTER

A s described thus far, doubles is a game of angles, anticipation, strategy, positioning, commitment, and communication. It is also a visual game! With good technique, footwork, position, skills, and opportunity you can still "blow it" by not looking at the ball completely or correctly you are attempting to strike. You can be more mentally focused on the detailed mechanics of _how_ to execute that shot or more focused on the desired target for your shot or watching what the other players are doing prior to hitting your current shot. In other words, we tend to take the ball for granted by not giving the BALL the visual commitment, attention, focus, detail, spacing and concentration it needs for you to be successful in that moment.

Honestly, I see this lack of focus on the ball too often in my own play when transitioning from lessons to real play, and in the play of many recreational players. As a teaching pro, my eyes tend not to be intently focused on the ball while hitting or feeding to enable more focus on my students. This regimented teaching habit works much of the time because I have hit a million plus balls, and my hand eye coordination is rather good especially when contacting slower moving balls such as feeds or just putting the ball back into play with certain students. However, when I am engaged in hitting with another pro or advanced level player who hits heavy- harder with lots of spin, I must **make** my eyes **commit** and **stay** on the incoming ball at contact. I share this occupational challenge, so you know that I am aware of your frustration and pain related to seeing the ball!

Often, an excellent opportunity to make an easy "put away" shot is blown due to a lack of focus on the ball. It seems the easier the shot there is a tendency to glance away from the ball, and the more challenging the shot the better the focus. This means the more time you have to make contact, the more thinking, options and glancing away. To think of the ball as your friend is a great idea to maintain a positive relationship with it, so you pay better attention to it than calling it negative names. You need the ball to work for you by making it do exactly what you want it to do. That success depends on how well you see the ball. Let's examine and discuss a few details about ball basics.

Most adult recreational players play with type 2 regulation tennis balls that are "optic yellow" with an official diameter of 6.54–6.86 cm (2.57–2.70 inches) as defined by the International Tennis Federation-ITF. [6] In addition, balls must have masses in the range of 56.0–59.4 g (1.97–2.09 ounces). [6] However, based on the player's skills, the ball can have a variety of spin, speed, and trajectories as it leaves the hitter's racquet and moves across the net that can make it easy or more challenging to see, contact and return.

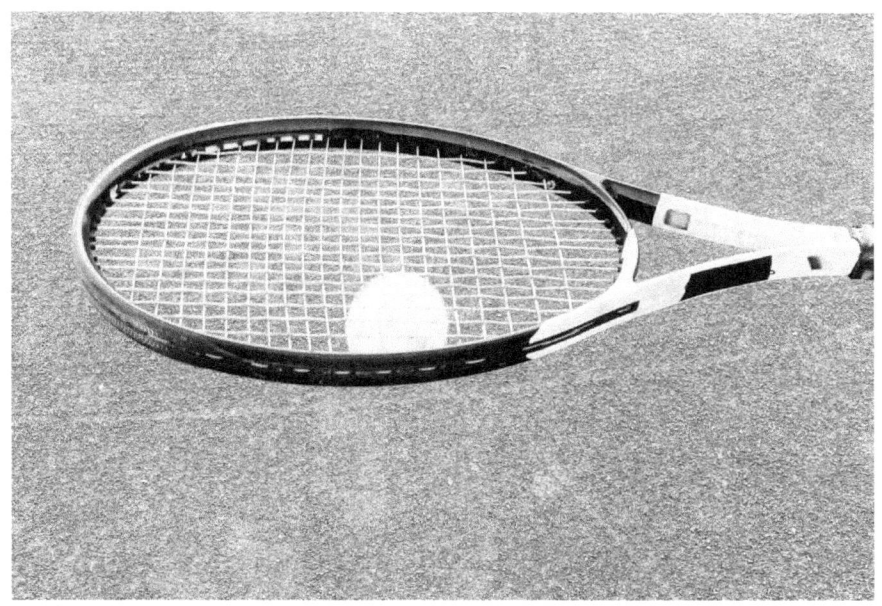

Image 8.1 shows racquet strings on top of the ball for bouncing down.

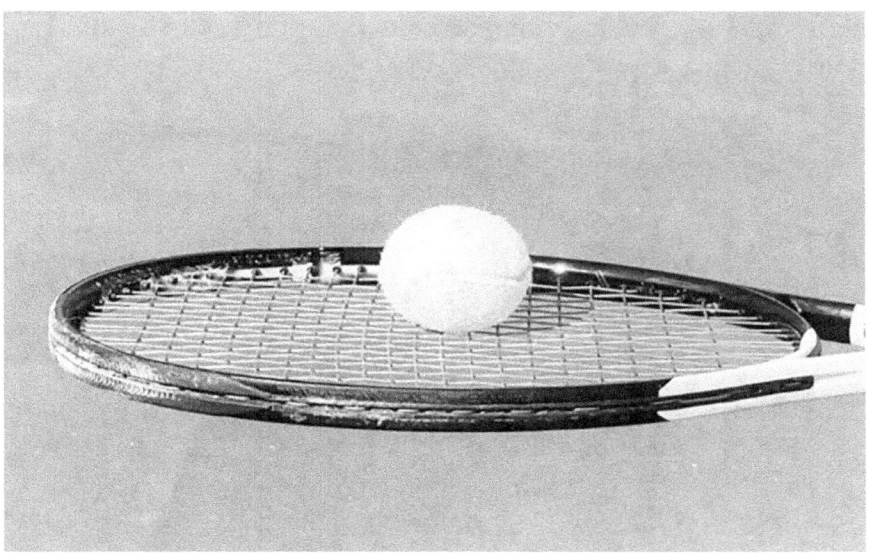

Image 8.2 shows racquet strings on the bottom or underneath the ball for bouncing up.

A good place to start to regain your confidence or training at seeing the ball better and making the ball obey your racquet face and intentions is to do ups and downs. As you can see in image 8.1, tapping the top of the ball with my racquet face will make the ball only go DOWN. Also, when your racquet face is underneath the ball tapping up on the bottom of the ball, it can only go UP. While doing these simple exercises for at least 10-20 bounces notice the brand of the ball, notice the fuzz and the white seams as in the details of the ball. These ups and downs should ideally be centered on your racquet face known as your sweet spot. Therefore, you are seeking to hit or strike most of your balls, shots, and strokes on your sweet spot. Where your sweet spot area connects with the ball is your *strike point.* In the following illustrations, I use the term *strike point* to enhance your detailed focus on the ball and your directional intent.

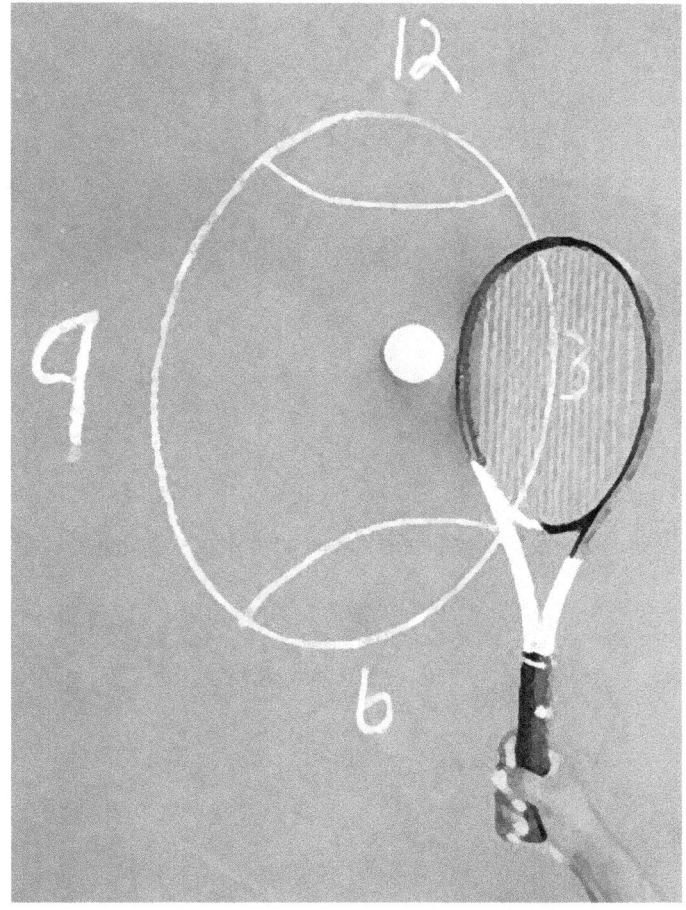

Image 8.3 shows an example of a 3 o'clock strike point.

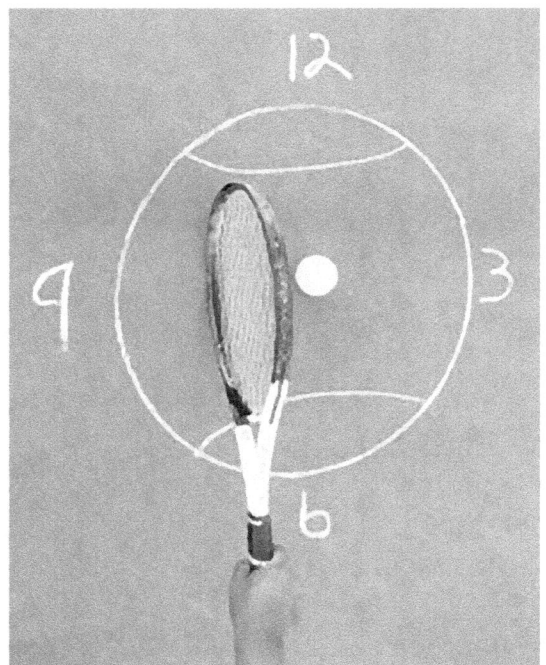

Image 8.4 shows an example of a 9 o'clock strike point.

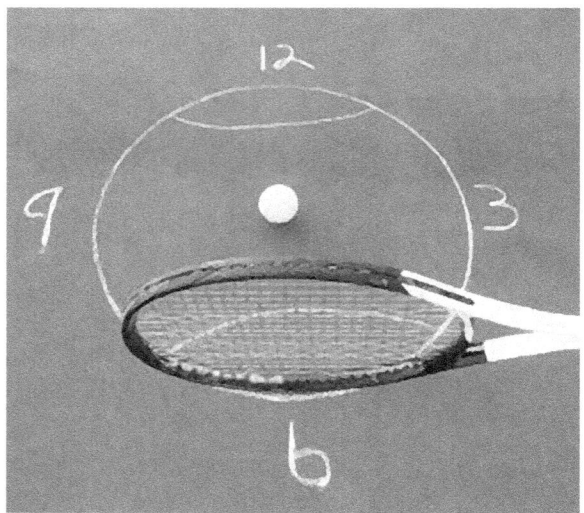

Image 8.5 shows an example of a 6 o'clock strike point.

In addition, if you strike the outer right side of the ball at 3 o'clock, it can only go in one direction, and striking it at 9 o'clock makes it go in the opposite direction as shown in image 8.3 and 8.4. These sample strike points will send the ball directly to the east or west to the next court or fence on a properly north and south facing court. Also, striking the ball at or near 6 o'clock will make the ball go straight with a follow through up to 12 as illustrated in image 8.5. Therefore, if you can see and focus on the sides of the ball—top, bottom or underneath, center or middle, left, right—you will better establish a visual and physical *strike point* on the ball.

I often share with my students, "the ball goes where you direct it" with your racquet from your *strike point*- A- to your intended target- B. If you can draw a straight line with a pencil on a piece of paper you can hit anywhere on the court, if you focus and commit your eyes to the correct *strike point* on the ball. In other words, when your pencil that is controlled by your hand makes a dot or period you can create whatever you desire from that dot-*strike point*. With NO commitment or intentions to what you want makes it harder to hit specific shots- lobs, CC FHs, CC BHs, volleys/OHs to the middle or down the line returns.

Profoundly, as you are hitting the ball at a particular *strike point* for a particular shot your eyes must remain on the ball at contact. After your finish or follow through you can look, focus, and track how and where the ball is going relative to your target B. At contact target B is a mental image. In other words, you cannot look at your physical target B while striking the ball. You must trust your mental imagery of the physical tennis court, your hitting location, and know exactly where you want to direct the ball. Also, the court is the same on the other side. For example, when putting in golf your eyes are down and focused on the ball at impact NOT on the hole. You know where the hole is after a few looks. Let's dig into my favorite tools to help you focus on the ball better to hit more shots where you INTEND!

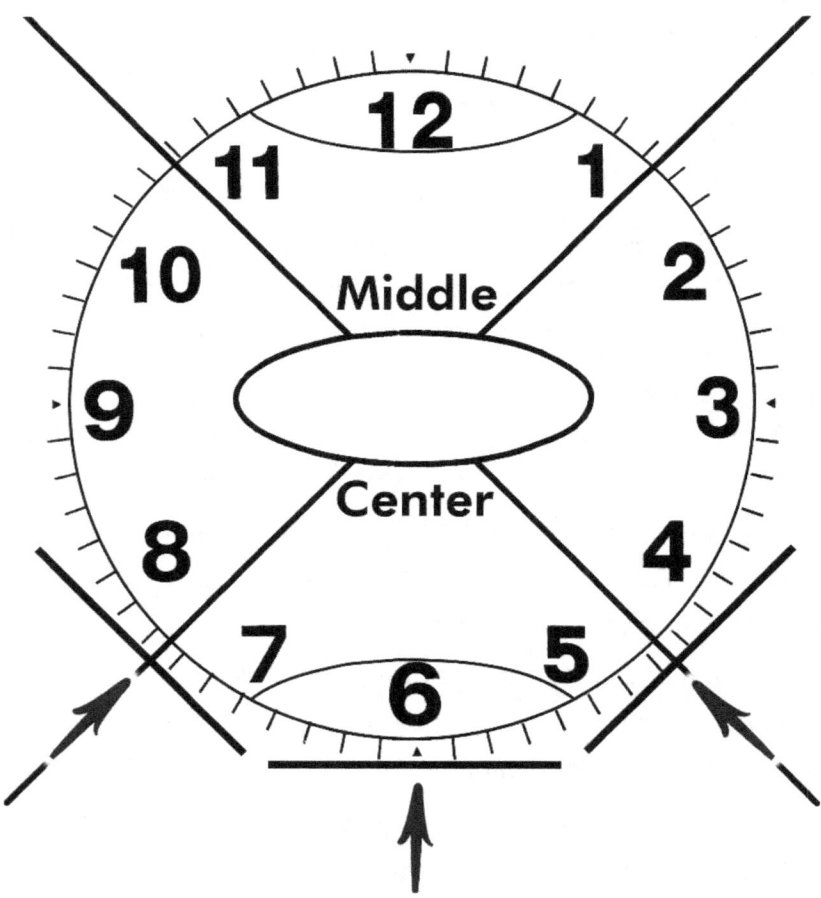

Image 8.6 shows a tennis ball as a clock.

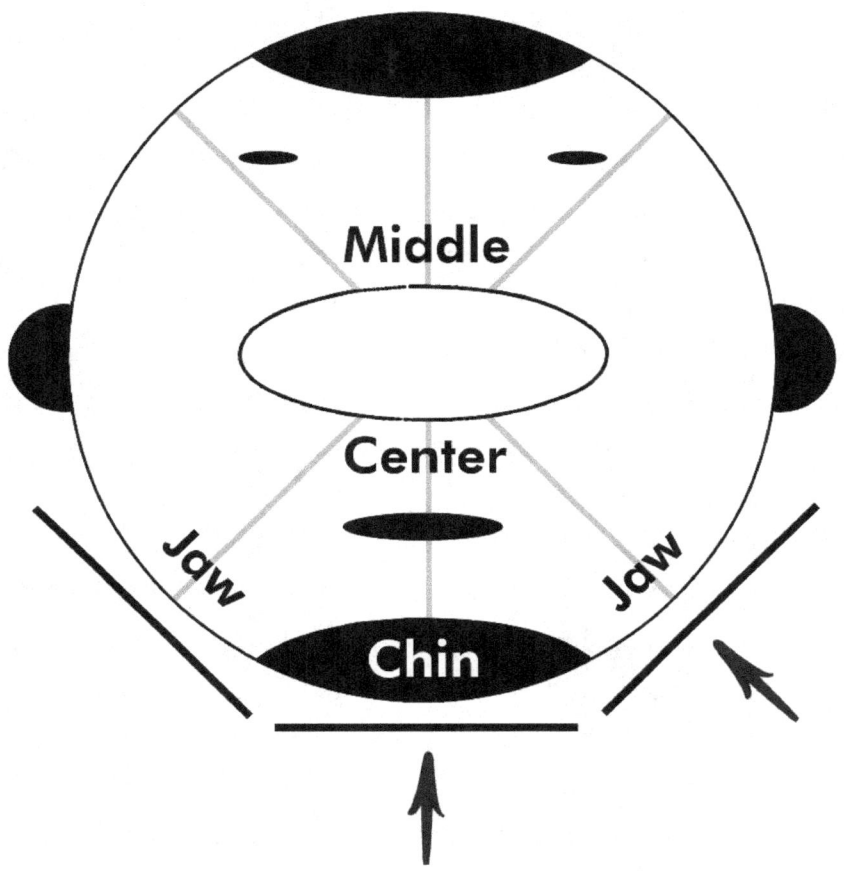

Image 8.6, continued, shows a tennis ball as a face.

As you know in doubles play, if you do not keep the ball away from the net player when hitting from the baseline, you are enabling your opponent's success and making it harder for you to win. At certain levels, I see too many balls floating up the middle or wrongly going straight towards the opposing net player in good position- ***High You Die***. As a correction, I suggest to the deep player to hit, strike the ball at 4 o'clock or 5 o'clock to create more cross court angle away from the net player with a FH or left-handed BH from the deuce court. Also, to hit more angle from the ad side with your BH or left- handed FH, you must strike the ball at 7 o'clock to 8 o'clock. If you intend to drive to your alley, straight or lob your *strike point* on the ball is closer to 6 o'clock-the center or bottom of the ball to make it go straight instead of cross court. Image 8.6 shows specific times that relate to specific strike points for cross court shots, lobs, and straight-ahead targets. Every time you want the ball to go straight or anywhere your *strike point* must be generally correct. Hitting the middle or center of the ball from the baseline or mid court would create a lower trajectory at the net and likely a shorter landing ball known as a FLAT ball or shot.

To hit deeper or "heavier" topspin groundstrokes, I always tell my students when hitting from the baseline or midcourt to hit or lift from the chin of the ball. *Hit on the Chin*! When hitting/lifting from the chin you will get more topspin. More spin means more balls IN. At times for specific shots such as slice groundstrokes, approach shots, drops, and short to short shots you will strike higher on the ball above the center to generate slice spin or to forcefully hit down on the ball for a put away shot. In addition, there is a left, right and center of the chin. When hitting cross court your *strike point* is either a left or right chin/jaw depending on how much angle you need. The popular and effective inside out righty FH from the ad or the inside out lefty FH from the deuce are excellent examples. As described, another perspective and option to see the ball better and commit to specific strike points for your desired shots, is to see the ball as a friendly face as illustrated in image 8.6.

As you know the ball has a label and seams to potentially help notice detail on the ball, but if the ball is traveling or rotating quickly with slice or topspin those white seams and label are not noticeable. To maximize your fun while playing tennis, I remind students that the ball is your friend, and it will do what you tell it with practice, intention, and commitment by striking it at specific points for your desired shot. Therefore, you must know exactly what shot you want and commit to it. If you see the ball as a smiling face or as a clock and commit your eyes to the correct strike point instead of just swinging at a yellow ball, you will have more success hitting where you want the ball to go such as: cross court, down the line, down the middle, higher or lower over the net. In addition, these strike points in general apply to all placed/aimed shots including volleys, overheads and serves. As mentioned, the ball goes where you direct it with your hand and racquet face from your *strike point*! For example, to place more FH and BH volleys and overheads accurately to the middle you are either striking the outside or inside of the ball not the middle or center of the ball. Striking near the center or middle of the ball at net will make the ball go straight back in play to the deep player in a one up and one back situation or towards an opposing net player's doubles alley or middle alley for a *One and Done or High You Die*. Also, during a deep to deep warm up from the baseline when hitting groundstrokes back and forth on the same half of the court you must hit more of the back of the ball (middle or bottom) to return the ball directly to the other player. Otherwise, hitting more on the inside or outside will make the ball go crosscourt and interrupt the other hitters on the other half.

Based on your situation/location and your intentions, if you know before striking what specific shot you want, you can commit to the appropriate *strike point* on the ball to make it happen. As stated, too many balls hit towards the opposing net player from your baseline area is bad for you and your partner at net. Your *Deep to Deep* shots need to go cross court with more angle (outside or inside strike point) or over the net player's head. Making this visual and mental commitment will build your confidence and trust in your abilities on the court with some regular practice. In match play or when playing points/games thinking about the mechanics of how to hit a specific shot or stroke can create a distraction from *where your racquet face needs to be to strike the ball for your desired result*. At some point you KNOW and *understand* how to hit a stroke or specific shot. This over thinking and obsessing tendency about your mechanics can get in the way of playing, not practicing, your best tennis when it really matters. To develop more confidence and consistency, the **BALL** needs your *attention* and *focus* at contact to execute more of your specific intentions. In addition, your eyes help you anticipate how the ball is coming back from the other side of the net. A deliberate focus on the bounce of the ball in front of you when at the net especially prior to their contact enables you to better anticipate how the ball is coming back. This focus on the bounce and strike allows you to track the ball early and prepare for your next shot before the ball gets to your side of the net. Also, before the ball bounces and even at their ***strike point*** you can indirectly notice or sense their comfort level as in struggling or not. Relative to the net height the ball has a low, medium, or high trajectory to help you anticipate how the ball is coming towards you when positioned at the net or the baseline. Because of your anticipation you can better plan, react, commit, and execute more quality shots with ***Happy Feet***.

To be clear when the ball reaches your side of the net, seeing the ball completely and knowing/committing where you intend to strike the ball for your desired shot is your top priority. Based on your situation and location always hit the high percentage shot as in the smart shot (***DSW***) unless you can afford the risk given the score or situation. When the ball is in front of you across the net, you can notice other things prior to or at contact such as their balance, timing/spacing and situation. Their strike point (inside, outside, center, underneath) tells you *where* the ball should go. Their spacing/timing (comfortable, early, late), swing type (big or small loop, straight back or short backswing), and situation (offense, defense, NML, good or bad position) should tell you *how* (fast, slow, low, high) the ball is coming towards you. Your eyes, feet and hands are your major assets on the court. For more confidence and trust in your strokes and shot making ability please continue to the next chapter!

SMART DOUBLES

CHAPTER 9

PRACTICE AND CLINICS:
OTHER FUN FORMS OF DOUBLES

P ractice sessions, lessons and clinics are better opportunities to think about and focus on one or two aspects of your mechanics related to HOW to hit certain strokes and specific shots. You may want more spin, angle, power, depth, or consistency. In this learning and reinforcing environment you can program your body with repetition and focus to hit the ball as desired. Several of your senses are in play such as sound, feel and sight. Not just thinking! At impact, the ball makes a certain sound and feels a certain way. At the net, the ball is traveling at a certain level or trajectory over the net as in high, medium, or low. You can change that trajectory by doing certain things. An awareness through all your senses of the details of your mechanics (grips, backswing, timing, contact, spacing, balance, follow through) when in the *practice mode* is beneficial! When in the *playing mode* for competition your focus is different, and you must use and trust your strengths and abilities you currently have NOT those shots and abilities you want in the future. Also, in the *playing mode* you must be aware of your opponent's tendencies, how they tend to strike the ball, how they move, and what type of balls/shots they prefer to hit just to name a few. Being aware of certain details on the other side of the net about your opponents is important in this mode. Often your good shots will create defense and struggle from a player or your opponents that you can benefit from. When practicing your focus is largely you, your strokes, shots, and skills. For example, if you currently have an inconsistent serve, practice your toss or add more spin for consistency and confidence. If you have a weaker backhand hit more backhands to make it more consistent and dependable. Therefore, if you are playing a match that you would like to win or do well in, hit serves that you can get in consistently and move to your left if right-handed, to hit more forehands from the ad side. In other words, I suggest, make practice about practice and playing about using your strengths to create more success.

There is an inner game of tennis classically written about in his book, *The Inner Game of Tennis* by author, Tim Gallwey. I first read his book in the 80's and have glanced at it many times over four decades for reminders related to teaching, coaching, and playing. It is an excellent book about important aspects of life, not just tennis, and worth reading. Unfortunately, for many, <u>over</u> thinking, judging, criticizing, analyzing, and critiquing can overwhelm and paralyze your mind and energy thus preventing your natural abilities to assist you especially when playing a game or match. This over thinking about what you already know can hinder your focus on the ball and your ability to make your desired shot. Also, negative energy for most of us gets in the way of playing our best to create and allow the desired outcome. Practice and practice with a smile for the skills and confidence you desire. In other words, try not to doubt yourself and your abilities. Focus on what you want and believe you can do it. With this book I seek to help make the ongoing process of learning, improving, and building your confidence at playing doubles easier, less complicated, so more players can enjoy and benefit from the game of doubles. One of my early tennis influencers- Arthur Ashe- was quoted saying: "Start where you are, use what you have, and do what you can."

From my experience it is more fun, beneficial, and effective to learn, sharpen and improve your *doubles specific skills* for competitive play in a small group of three or four similar players. In this small group environment, you can practice and reinforce your doubles related skills with an instructor or an advanced level player, meet other similar players to practice or play with, and share the cost. This type of lesson/clinic is a wonderful opportunity to see how other players hit, play, move, position, and to enjoy the social aspect of doubles. If you play mostly doubles it is ideal to grow and enhance your doubles specific skills in a doubles environment. If you play on a league team, you have access to players and hopefully a teaching pro/coach who can help you improve as a doubles player. It is ideal to find a few partners you enjoy playing with and to practice, drill, and take clinics/lessons with them to enhance your partnership potential and match play experience. It can be more challenging to enjoy doubles even just for fun with a variety of random partners.

The challenging and fun journey of learning, developing, and improving your strokes- FH, BH, serve, OH and volleys, can be shared with others including the cost. Depending on where you live, I recommend that you find and enroll in weekly or regular "stroke clinics" for beginners, advanced beginners, and intermediate players to first learn or improve your basic strokes and skills. You may be athletic, played sports in the past and can hit hard, but most of your shots go out or into the net. Perhaps you did not play sports previously but now you have the time and resources to enjoy tennis. Establishing control and consistency with variations of speed, spin and height over the net is important to get more balls in and enjoy the game. Many public facilities, swim-tennis communities and private clubs offer group clinics that will help improve and reinforce your developing strokes and mechanics. These facilities that offer regular instructional programs often include round robins in which you can practice and reinforce your skills and meet other similar players. Guess what type of tennis is usually played at these events? Yes, doubles! At some point you must learn how to play Smart Doubles®!

Not all advanced players or high-level players can teach or want to teach, and not all teaching pros are outstanding for everyone. Most certified teaching professionals do a respectable job working with recreational players-beginners, advanced beginners, intermediate and advanced players. However, our playing and teaching backgrounds, training, education, and experience do vary, and our personalities and communication skills vary as well. Working with a professional instructor or advanced player is beneficial if you have access to someone. In the absence of formal training and instructors there are other creative options to help improve your skills on your own or with a friend. For example, with two or three players you can practice hitting cross court groundstrokes and playing cross court points with or without a serve. The more balls you can keep in play cross court the more points you can win in a match with patience and consistency. Also, with two players you can use only the left or right half of the court including the doubles alley to practice keeping the ball in play, lobbing over an imaginary net player, and hitting down the middle alley or the doubles alley. As you know, often doubles is played two back and when you are in a deep position hitting deep is your best option. Another option is to practice, hit or play out points two against one. With another player or two you have many creative options to build your consistency and confidence, have fun, and obtain exercise. It seems that millions of prospective players and current players worldwide are interested in learning and improving at tennis, but many are largely self-taught for various reasons. In this book, I support and encourage self-initiated ways to learn and grow your skills.

Being curious about tennis in general or a student of the game is an ongoing process, but with access to the internet you can conveniently find tennis resources. You can learn about stroke mechanics by watching online videos, reading books, and watching others play. However, do not become overwhelmed or intimidated by advice, styles, and techniques that are perhaps too challenging or complicated for you. Initially, your objective from instruction is to learn the basics as in how to stroke the ball that create a foundation for your skills. Try not to focus on what other popular ATP/WTA playing professionals do. For starters, you want simple progressions that enable you to make contact, direct the ball with spin where you want, and to keep the ball in play for consistency. Always use common sense and acknowledge what feels right for you. To hit and play like a pro means doing the basics well with many years of practice and experience. A high-level player's style, look, motion, grips, and strokes are unique to her and so are yours. By watching advanced level players, you can certainly reinforce the basics, and see how and why they are winning or losing points, games, and matches.

In addition, you can rent a ball machine at a facility or purchase one for yourself. You can even *share* the hourly rental fee or purchase price of a machine with another player or players. Practicing with a ball machine on a court is a fantastic way to feel like you are playing tennis while improving your strokes and consistency. You can practice patterns and hitting specific shots including volleys and groundstrokes to specific targets. Depending on the machine, you may have more options for what you can do with a ball machine to accelerate your skills, growth, and confidence. Please use good balls not dead balls when using the ball machine. As stated, if possible, share the cost of a good machine with a few other local players to help make it feasible to practice and build your skills. Hit lots of balls and make it fun!

One of my favorite low-cost, very consistent, and responsive practice options is to hit balls against a concrete wall. Hitting against the wall is a terrific way to practice by hitting hundreds of balls with good technique, good contact space/area, and strike point on the ball. To practice your *deep to deep* groundstrokes, stand 30-40 feet away from the wall to rally at 3-6 feet above an imaginary net. Since the wall is so responsive, I recommend using used balls, not new, for hitting against the wall. Also, to get started, you can drop hit each ball one at a time to get used to how the ball comes back based on how hard you hit and where the ball hits against the wall. Then progress to letting one ball bounce twice between shots until you can better control how the ball comes back to hit with only one bounce. Be patient as you obtain a feel for how to hit against the wall.

Hitting on the wall is great cardio exercise and natural footwork practice simultaneously in a short period of time. Also, hitting against the wall can accelerate the development of your skills. The more you use it the better you become. By hitting 5, 10, 15, 20, 25 FHs or BHs in a row straight to the wall builds consistency and confidence. Striking the ball at 6 o'clock with a low to high or lifting swing from the chin for topspin is ideal. As stated, if you can hit straight, you can hit anywhere. During your rallies if the ball bounces twice, no biggie, keep going. After warming up for a few minutes, hit all forehands to a certain number, and then all backhands to a certain number. Also, you can practice your topspin and slice strokes *deep to deep* farther away from the wall. When closer to the wall you can practice short and transition shots with less pace as in slices and drops. Basically, the ball comes from the wall the way you send it as in high, low, fast, and slow. The ball is returned from the wall quicker than usual because it does not travel to the other baseline when hitting on a full court. In other words, you have less time in between shots when hitting against the wall. Therefore, anticipate how the ball is coming back from the wall and prepare quickly for the next approaching ball.

In addition, hitting against a wall is a fantastic way to develop more consistency in less time since the wall does not miss unless it contains holes or cracks. Therefore, you should become more consistent the more you use the wall. The wall will provide instant feedback based on how and where you hit, but it will not provide verbal instruction. However, it does indicate how you hit each ball based on how it returns from the wall. You are learning, feeling, reinforcing, and growing on your own. Ideally, you want the ball to come right back to you so you can hit repeatedly with one bounce without struggle. You want to obtain a good, simple, and natural rhythm on the wall. Depending on their level, it may be challenging to obtain a similar good hitting rhythm with another player or two. The wall is very consistent once the ball reaches the wall. After 30-60 mins of this type of practice session you may get bored, but it really works when used on a regular basis to expedite and facilitate development of your control, spacing-contact area-consistency, and confidence. Your first time practicing on the wall may be awkward or challenging, but you will improve quickly if you return and keep trying. Try to maintain a good contact area/space slightly in front of your body. Your contact area is where you contact the ball in relation to your body. It is the space between you and the ball.

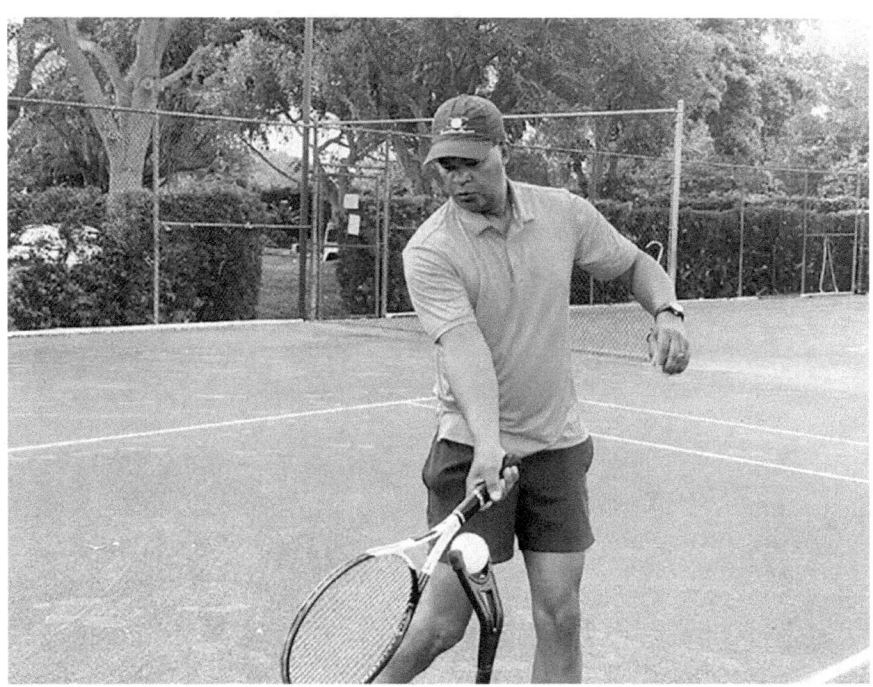

Image 9.1 shows FH lifting from 6 o'clock strike point or near the center of the chin with good contact spacing.

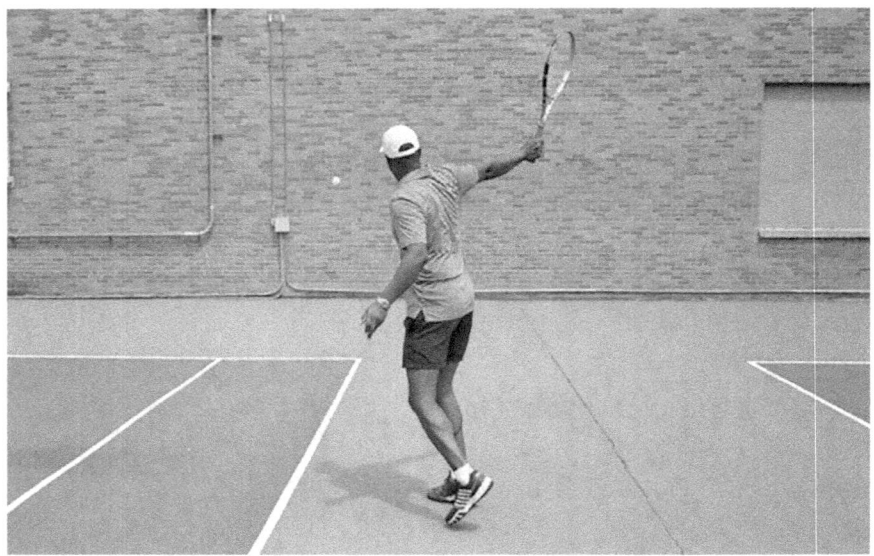

Image 9.2 shows BH hit from 6 o'clock area or
center of the chin to make the ball go straight and return to me.

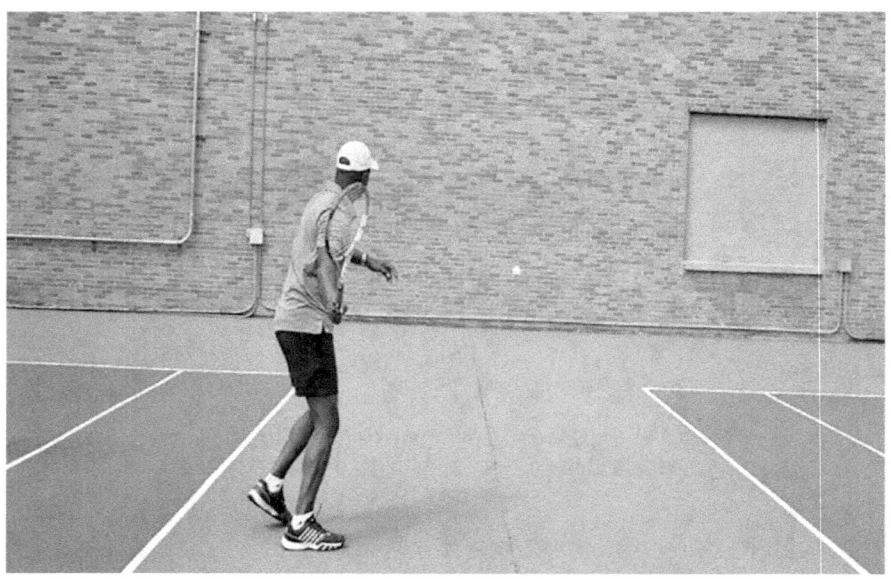

Image 9.3 shows FH hit straight to the wall with 6 o'clock or
center of the chin strike point for top spin.

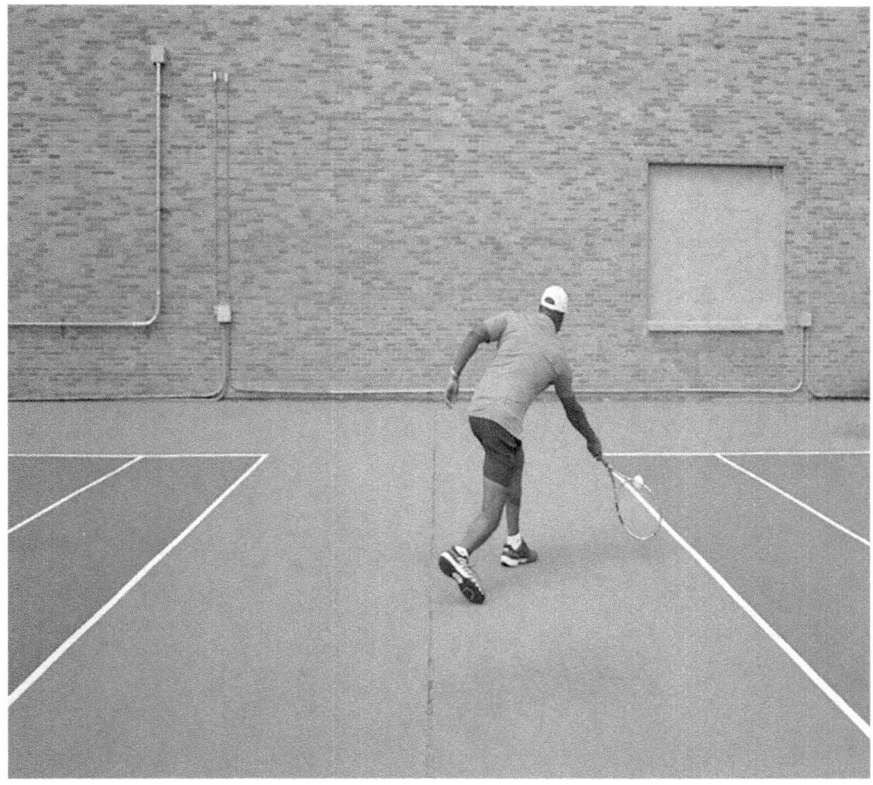

Image 9.4 shows an example of struggling to hit a low FH.

Depending on where you live, your resources and level of interest in playing tennis, you may or may not have access to formal or organized tennis. There are many seasonal, recreational, random, off the radar and fringe players who are largely self-taught. These players or interested players may not "belong" to or have access to an organization or facility. Therefore, being open and creative to find tennis opportunities and other interested players may take some effort. Usually, high schools have tennis courts where you may find a wall and the opportunity to practice and play. As a teenager, I hit against the wall for practice almost daily. As an adult, occasionally I use the wall to warm up and practice. In my next book, *The Enrichment of Life Begins with Love*, I will share how regularly hitting the wall over several years as a teen profoundly impacted my life and career.

CHAPTER 10

WINNING, LOSING, LEARNING, FUN: ALL GOOD

Upon relocating from Little Rock, AR to Atlanta, GA in 1993 to work as a teaching pro, I was focused largely on and more experienced at working with advanced juniors. After working for a year for two junior academies- Norman Wilkerson and Ralston Gorman Academy- I landed my first director's job in 1994 at Tucker Racquet Club. Instantly, my focus changed to working with the club's 6-8 adult league teams that participated in a very popular metro wide league known as ALTA. This enormous and very popular adult and junior league had approximately 80k participants at that time. [1]

In the spring of 1995, our C-6 weekday ladies team won the ALTA City Championship. Instantly, my passion for coaching doubles teams was born! This was a significant accomplishment for this hardworking group of ladies and a significant accomplishment for me, especially being new at this club and to Atlanta. In addition, while in my early 30's, I began playing doubles in the Men's AA1 division ALTA team tennis league amongst other teaching pros, former collegiate players, and touring pros. It was new, fun, competitive and exciting. Being an active competitive doubles player freshly reinforced several important teachable concepts for my teams. In my view, Atlanta was and still is Tennis Town USA. During my 11 years of working in Atlanta in the public, private and residential sectors as both an employee and independent contractor, I gave thousands of doubles strategy and positioning clinics and watched hundreds of league team matches at all levels. By watching my teams play competitive matches, made me keenly aware of why certain teams and partnerships won and lost matches.

Observing the weekday ladies' home matches on Thursday mornings and the businesswomen's matches on Sundays was a no brainer. In ALTA, the home team customarily provided light snacks, appetizers, and beverages to share with the visiting team. Many of my ladies' teams took pride in their table presentation and snack/food choices. Usually, the food was homemade and delicious! The men's teams that I coached and played on played their matches on Saturday mornings at 9am and usually provided doughnuts, chips, nuts, water, and beer to share with their away team. The snacks/food and beverage options were typically quite different depending on where and who was playing. Nevertheless, as a coach, it was my perspective and job to help my teams and partnerships be successful on game day. Observing match play on game day compared to just conducting clinics was instrumental for me as a coach.

Winning, especially at doubles requires many things, but as you know you cannot win all the time. However, you can always put forth your best effort, learn and grow from losses if you and your partner talk and reflect, especially after a match. Each match is won or lost for specific reasons. Your coach can provide helpful feedback, explain why you won or did not win and provide good partnership options and suggestions. It is helpful to know what you could have done differently against the two players you just lost to. Also, it is greatly beneficial to acknowledge what you did well that contributed to your win. When partners do not talk about certain things before, during and after a match, you make it harder to play Smart Doubles®. When your pro/coach watches you play, he can better coach you and develop drills that will help reinforce your strengths and improve your weaknesses. In fact, pay your coach or an assistant to watch a few of your important matches. In addition, supervised match play and round robins that are watched by your coach are excellent opportunities for him to help you play smarter and position properly- Smart Doubles®. As you know, practice and match play are different. Often, the difference between the two are focus, communication, determination, and commitment.

Patience pays! Rushing the situation, getting in a hurry, and trying to be a hero tends to produce more unforced errors and low percentage shots. Also, overhitting tends to create more unforced errors. Often, finesse is best. If you are struggling just put the ball back in play or lob. When positioned in the deep court it is especially important that you hit *deep to deep*. Be patient and rally cross court away from the net player. The lob is an excellent *deep to deep* shot in the one up and one back formation. It is often underused and overused at times at the risk of being too predictable. If two players are playing two back, you can drive deep to the middle to see how they manage that area. Often, they will struggle deciding quickly who hits the middle ball. As discussed, lobbing over the opposing net player especially from the deuce court is an outstanding tactic. This shot makes a righty travel over to the ad court forcing a switch to retrieve a lob with a BH. Most often, that is a tough situation for the team switching by chasing down a lob. Practice and use the lob more often as one of your *deep to deep* options especially on deuce court points or when a lefty is serving or receiving on the ad side. Do not give points away! Be patient and minimize your unforced errors, especially when deep in the back court!

Finish the point at the net! To help your partner hold serve and to break serve more often, you must poach, fake poach, distract, and create subtle chaos to obtain more finishing volleys and overheads. It is imperative that you *"Follow the Ball"* to better position closer to where the ball lands or is being hit from to intercept the likely trajectory as in cross court or up for a lob. At the net see where and how the ball bounces and move a step or two towards the ball before the contact. Show your *happy feet* to make them notice you more than the ball or their best shot opportunity. When they commit with their swing especially from a deep location or a struggling situation you can commit to intercept with ***Happy Feet***. Often it will take two shots at net to finish the point as in your first volley followed by your second volley or OH because you are following the ball and your shot. If you hit a good volley at net to the middle, ***FTB*** to reposition for the finishing shot. Middle then alley is an excellent combo of shots at the net, and often the second volley/shot can be a finessed short angle instead of a power ball especially if your middle shot forces either the deep player or net player out of position.

For example, if the serve or groundstroke shot lands in the middle of the court, FTB to the middle. Your improved position may provide an opportunity to angle the ball wide off the court away from the deep player or towards the opposing net player. For example, if moving to the right, hit to your right towards the middle, or net player's feet or the alley you are moving towards. Occasionally, when moving to your left or right towards the center of the court to hit a volley, you may be able to angle the ball short off the court behind or opposite your momentum. For example, this situation often occurs when finishing the point with a second shot that is defensively returned from the middle from either the out of position net player or deep player. Also, when you are close to the net and moving left or right striking a sitter or high ball, it makes sense to angle the ball short and wide to the alley you are leaving. However, this shot attempt and situation may provide an opportunity for the deep player to exploit your alley if the shot is not hit perfectly. Moving left or right towards the middle of the court will create opportunities to finish the point wide to either alley depending on your position or movement and where the ball is relative to the net. Usually, when in a good position, hitting in front of your movement is a high percentage opportunity to finish the point.

In addition, during a cross court rally, when the ball bounces wide in the alley in front of you, you must cover some of your alley enough to force the return more to the middle or cross court of which you are partially responsible for too. Be ready to cover at least two steps towards the middle while covering your alley. More balls will travel CC than down your wide alley. When you see your opponent struggling in a deep position or near the service line you should anticipate a likely CC attempt with a *Low You Go*.

Everyone has a different reach and reaction time. If your feet are not happy and noisy at the net, you are not a threat. Finally, with great position do not put the ball back in play when you can put it away to the middle or alley! Being in good position at the net enables well placed volleys and overheads with purpose. Mirage, one of my Longboat Key colleagues for many years likes, "stick it and defend it" If you stick or place a volley or OH to the middle you must "pinch" (FTB) the middle to anticipate another shot if the ball comes back. Finishing the point, game, or match with a volley or OH is great fun!

Make a plan! Get your serve inside the box to the middle. Move left or right to hit more of the shots/returns you want. Play two back. Do the Australian on the ad side or deuce if the lefty is serving. Keep the ball away from the best player. Control the net if invited consistently with short balls. Lob to force a switch and struggle. Do not sit in NML. Either move up to volley or move back to hit groundstrokes. If something is not working, change. Share your observations about your opponents, strategic ideas, and tactics before, in between points or when changing sides. If your partner does not like to talk strategy, situations, and tactics, find another partner if you prefer to win more matches than lose. Doubles is a partnership that requires simple, effective communication depending on the level of play. *No plan is a losing strategy*!

Get your first serve in! Too many recreational players overhit their first serve that has little to no chance of going in. Then their second serve is a softy that enables the returner to be more aggressive. Learn and regularly practice a medium serve that goes in first and more often. As you toss and before you swing, you should acknowledge a good or bad ball toss. Focus on the correct toss and be patient. Do not chase or force the obvious bad toss that is behind you, too low, or too far out in front, or left or right. In this muscle memory creating situation you want to reinforce more of what you want, NOT what you do not want. If the toss is not what you want- *LIG!* For your recreational games and matches there is no limit on your tosses. Being patient is good practice for the returner too. The more serves that are placed in play, the more your partner can contribute to helping you win your service game. If you cannot get your serve in, you cannot win! In match play Double faults are gifts to the other team. Give the returner something to hit or miss, not free points!

Play defense when the ball is behind you! When at the net there are basically two modes of doubles-offense and defense. Too often players stay in the offensive mode and position when their partner is hitting from behind them. When the ball zings by you at the net in good position, you must quickly move back-**Tennis Two Step** to play defense and cover some of the middle. In the one up and one back formation, when the ball goes *back* you move *back* and focus on the opposing net player. Quickly glancing back at your partner to see where they are or what they are doing or likely to do is necessary during their times of struggle. A lob over your head at net is a good example after you switch sides. Another situation for a quick look back is a wide or short ball that is challenging for them to return. In this back or defensive position, you are protecting yourself and MORE of the middle. When the ball clears the opposing net player-green light, you move *forward/up* to offense again towards the bounce of the ball-**FTB**. This up and back flow is what I call the **Tennis Two Step** that you do at net every time when the ball passes by you cross court or over you as in a deep lob or back to your deep partner. To keep it simple, up for offense and back for defense! The up and offensive position is where you can start when your partner is serving. Therefore, as an SP you are in the *driver's seat* to start the point. If there is an opposing net player, you must move back two steps to the *back seat* for defense. After moving back, if you do not move up again once the ball clears the opposing net player, you may struggle hitting an offensive volley if your opponent hits low at or near you. If most of your points on both sides of the net are played in the one up and one back formation, you must move back to play defense. When you have two players up against you alone at the net, you are likely in the defensive mode until your partner hits a perfect low or high ball that allows you to move forward. I heard defense wins championships!

Adjust! Too often, net players position too close to the net as if their opponents are going to place the ball directly to their racquet to slam. Being too close to the net makes it easier for a lob to go over your head. Also, if your partner from their deep position hits straight or near the opposing net player when you are positioned too close to the net, the middle between you and your partner is wide open. ***Money Middle***! When back for defense, your focus is the opposing net player, not your partner. If you look back too often or for too long, you have no idea what is going on in front of you. During a ***Deep to Deep*** rally, you will know if you need to move back even more by watching the movement of the other net guy especially if he is moving towards the net or the ball or if their racquet goes up for an overhead. Also, when playing against frequent lobbers, you can play slightly deeper than usual at the net to hit overheads or move back to the baseline to take their lob over your head away completely. Certain players hit higher, lofty balls with less pace that make it easier for others to hit lobs. This may place a hardship on the back player by forcing them to switch too often. In this situation, playing two back will neutralize the lob and allow both players to share more shots from the baseline. A lefty on the deuce who may be serving and a righty on the ad side both positioned back may be a good opportunity to hit more forehands from the middle.

As a reminder when you are the SP, your default position at net should be at least halfway between the net and the service line or slightly inside that imaginary halfway line. This position is ideal for the typical or average recreational player. From this location you can direct offensive volleys with contact above the net level and move back a few steps to take more overheads than switching. During a cross court rally, if you are out of position as in up when you should be back, you are making it easier for the other net player to target you and especially the middle- *One and Done*! If you do not move up for offense and back for defense, you will likely lose and struggle because of poor positioning. Once the ball clears the opposing net player's racquet, you can move up to offense because you know where the ball is going. In other words, you do not have to wait until the ball lands deep to move up to offense. At net, your job is to *Follow The Ball* up two steps and back two steps, until there is a reason to move back even more such as a deep lob behind you or wide angle that pulls your partner off the court. If you do not like to play at the net or are having a dreadful day at the net, you can stay back and play from the baseline. Another option is to stay up at the net and *practice* your Tennis Two Step, FTB and good positioning. When at the net you cannot stay in the same location/position. *Move it or lose it*!

Hit more high-percentage shots! Smart Doubles® features hitting more high-percentage shots based on your situation, position/location than low-percentage shots. Also, Smart Doubles® features being in the best position/location to play offense or defense. In supervised match play, round robins, and clinics your pro/coach can better coach you with your shot selection and positioning. As stated, when struggling put the ball back in play as best as you can. In doubles, there is *always* a middle between the two players. It is the opening, the hole and always a high-percentage shot in the offensive mode! When hitting from certain locations against certain formations, it is smart to hit to the middle. The ball hit to the middle tends not to come back since there is usually no racquet in the middle-**Money Middle**! Too many recreational players jump into league play, competitive doubles, or even social doubles without fully understanding and practicing the basic strategy, tactics, and proper positioning for playing Smart Doubles®. Do not try risky, difficult shots when out of position or struggling. By quickly acknowledging your situation, you can better commit to the ball and the right shot. The doubles game is simple with a limited number of situations and possibilities. Therefore, learn and play the game properly and keep it simple.

Learning is a huge part of playing and winning! Each practice session, match, casual/fun game, round robin, or stroke clinic is an opportunity to gain experience and grow your skills. Some people are extremely competitive, moderately competitive, and some are not competitive, so they say. Regardless of your skill level, you can play and enjoy doubles for fun even if you are not very fond of competition. Doing your best along with a partner provides an opportunity to enhance your skills, health, and lifestyle. Baby steps! Only a small percentage of young players relative to the entire population of players have a career playing tennis. For most of us, tennis is simply an activity for exercise, enjoyment, and comradery among other active people.

As you know and can see, the game of singles is vastly different compared to doubles. You are using the same strokes but in a unique way. Hitting the ball back and forth and covering the entire court for singles is certainly more exercise and challenge that require more skill, athleticism, consistency, determination, and focus. At least in doubles you only cover half the court with a partner to help and support you for the entire game. In fact, playing doubles can benefit your singles play if you desire to play singles. From my perspective, getting involved in any organized doubles activity is a win-win!

CHAPTER 11

CENTER STAGE FOR RECREATIONAL TENNIS: DOUBLES LEAGUES

Although we are entertained by grueling singles matches on television, off camera in our communities, recreational players play and enjoy mostly doubles. Upon visiting several busy facilities with programming, especially at prime time, you are most likely to see more courts being used for doubles play than singles. Doubles leagues and their participants are good sources of revenue for facilities and teaching pros. Regardless of your age and level you can enjoy the game of doubles on a formal or informal basis. Just getting out there with three or four players hitting balls, playing points, doing simple drills or exercises can be fun. Being a seasonal, occasional recreational player who enjoys playing on a casual basis can be great fun and exercise too. Obviously, playing more often creates additional benefits such as physical activity, meeting new people, fun, and growth. Depending on where you live you may have additional options to get more involved with specific forms of organized league play. Often, nearby facilities and communities will organize seasonal or year-round informal league play. Leagues come in a variety of formats for juniors and adults. Some leagues offer both singles and doubles, but more league participants play doubles. Recreational leagues are usually formatted based on level, age range, same gender as in men or ladies or coed.

To further enhance your growth and improvement at tennis you may have opportunities to participate in an organized city, county, or national league such as the USTA or Ultimate Tennis. With approximately 300,000 players participating nationally each year, the USTA League is currently the USA's single largest adult competitive tennis league. [14] Ultimate Tennis features a flex format that allows you to play based on your schedule with the same partner in mixed and regular doubles. According to their website, they have leagues available year-round currently in six states with approximately 85k members. [14] In addition, there is a T2Tennis League currently offered in Atlanta, Charlotte, and Denver. Their website says currently they have over 118,000 members. [10] Another fast-growing league option for adults and juniors is Universal Tennis that features flex leagues now available in more than 85 cities in the U.S., Canada, Mexico, Europe, and Australia. [13] Universal Tennis uses the UTR rating system that ranges from 1-16.5 that globally determines your level based on recent competitive play.

It seems ALTA is the largest metropolitan tennis league in the world with approximately 80k members. [1] If you live in the multi-county metro of Atlanta, you can participate in ALTA, USTA, T2Tennis, Ultimate Tennis, Universal Tennis leagues and others year-round. These leagues are available at a variety of public courts, parks, facilities, private clubs, and residential communities (apartments, condominiums, swim-tennis neighborhoods). The public tennis court accessibility and infrastructure in the Atlanta metro was developed and is supported by the surrounding municipalities. This maximizes the opportunity to play and enjoy tennis for the community at large. In addition, many residential communities are strategically developed to provide tennis amenities. Unless it is below 32 degrees or raining, a typical week including the weekend is composed of league tennis related activity such as regular matches, make up matches, team clinics, partnership lessons/ private clinics, practice matches and round robins. For 11 years I was fortunate to experience an enormous level of tennis activity in Tennis Town USA that was mostly driven by recreational players engaged in league doubles activity.

Florida is one of the best states in which to fully enjoy a lifestyle of outdoor activity year-round including tennis on soft and hard courts. Outdoor tennis courts provide an attractive amenity to a variety of neighborhoods, resorts, gated communities, and country clubs. In addition, it seems most municipalities in Florida provide public courts and parks for its local citizens and seasonal visitors to enjoy tennis through the public sector. I have enjoyed working on Longboat Key as a teaching pro since the fall of 2004. Teaching at the #1 rated Colony Beach & Tennis Resort as a staff professional was my first experience working in the hospitality sector. We mainly served hotel guests, seasonal unit owners and renters, and locals.

Since relocating to Florida, I must say that I have enjoyed working and playing almost exclusively on soft courts on our beautiful gulf coast. Longboat Key and Siesta Key are barrier islands that bring a few million visitors from all over the world especially during season from November through April. In addition, on Longboat Key we have many seasonal second homeowners who regularly enjoy this area as well and return to their regular homes for the summer and fall. In other words, the entire state of Florida including our Sarasota/ Bradenton/ Longboat Key area is home to many retirees and active sports enthusiasts!

I am certain the late Nick Bollettieri made this area more popular among the international tennis community with his innovative style of tennis leadership when he began as an instructor at the Colony Beach & Tennis Resort in 1978. Then in the early 80s, he opened the Nick Bollettieri Tennis Academy in Bradenton, FL a few miles away from Longboat Key, now known as the IMG Academy. Many current and former professional tennis players, former collegiate players and international coaches live and work on the gulf coast and throughout the state. Florida in general is a hot bed for high performance and professional level tennis training for the younger players as well as for adult recreational players who play competitively and just for fun. In Florida, there is an enormous level of recreational tennis activity that is showcased in at least one hundred unique localized recreational leagues mostly for doubles play. Since living and working in Florida,

I have a greater appreciation for competitive senior men's and women's tennis due to the quality and abundance of senior players from 50+ in Southwest Florida and in the entire state. It is nice to see both men and women players in their 50's, 60's, 70's, 80's and 90's competing and enjoying tennis. This reality and range in active players reinforces that tennis is an excellent activity for longevity regardless of when you begin.

In the Sarasota and Manatee County area we offer the Tri Cities Doubles League for ladies from October to mid-March. According to the current coordinator, Mel Howard, this league has approximately 2200 participants in their database from 3.0-4.5 across 32 facilities. For the men in our area, we play in the Suncoast Doubles League. According to the current president, Fred Budde and teammate, the Suncoast League has approximately 1400 active players across 40 clubs with 19 different divisions. In addition, we have USTA, Ultimate Tennis and Universal Tennis league options. In other nearby cities such as Tampa, Clearwater, St. Petersburg, Ft. Myers, Naples, and Orlando there are several other local unique league options. These leagues are unique to each area including age, level, availability of players and number of facilities. Depending on the area such as Tampa, there are more year-round residents and younger adult players. In more seasonal areas such as Longboat Key/Sarasota, you have a substantial number of seasonal players. Where you live will ultimately determine your league options.

Finding a facility, a team to play on, and a regular partner or partners are all potential challenges depending on where you live. Unfortunately, leagues may not be available in smaller cities and rural areas. My advice is to make some calls to local clubs/facilities, search online for local leagues in your area, or talk to other players to learn about facilities, courts, and opportunities near you. At tenniscores.com which is an online scoring and management system for recreational leagues, you can search for some, not all, available leagues in your city or nearby cities. This website seems to be an excellent tool especially if you are relocating. In addition, the Global Tennis Network can be a resource for finding courts, players and setting up your own leagues, ladders, and events.

It is exciting to know based on my recent research that there are thousands of localized and available league options with the flexibility to accommodate millions of recreational players at a variety of levels and locations worldwide. For younger and working players who need to play on the weekend or evenings, flex leagues provide a wonderful opportunity for those players with a busier lifestyle and schedule! It is important to think of the game of doubles, especially organized league doubles, as an opportunity to obtain regular exercise and meet other active, interesting people. However, you will meet people with lots of "attitude" and bad behavior that you do not care for at all. Occasionally, people will say and do things that are rude, inappropriate, inconsiderate, dishonest-cheating, and unsportsmanlike. Yes, there are players at all levels who need to win more than be honest about the score, line calls and their performance. This should not be a deal breaker not to compete or enjoy tennis. My comment serves as a reminder that there are all types of people, personalities, and players involved in the sport. Your coach, team captain or partner can assist you when your opponents or even a teammate is a sponsor of drama. Often these potential conflicts are petty or related to questionable line calls or simply a misunderstanding. At times, you need thick skin, the ability to be diplomatic and the willingness to take the high road. Your communication skills can be your most important asset both on and off the court! All of us are in communication-based partnerships unless you are incarcerated or deceased. Therefore, participating in the sport of tennis through a league is an opportunity to grow your game and enhance your lifestyle. It is a win- win!

As a head pro/director, I enjoyed being involved in the formation, maintenance and coaching of teams that played where I was employed. However, some teams and captains did not need or want my regular input. Captains are volunteers and need to be appreciated especially when they do an excellent job and make positive things happen for the benefit of the team. However, they are human- imperfect- and may not be a good fit for you or maybe the team. You may need to be patient and selective until you find the right team and place for your purpose, personality, and skills. In my opinion, it is important for teams to discuss and decide before the season starts to play their best available players to be more competitive or to play a random line up to include more available players on the team. When a team openly decides to play competitively-to win as many matches as possible- and play the best available players and partnerships, it creates more commitment, excitement, and potential success for the team. I believe most people would agree that playing on a winning team is more fun than playing on a losing team. Of course, this unified team position and understanding depends on the quantity and quality of your roster and the type of league. Certain leagues, teams and players are more competitive than others. Playing for fun is totally fine as in not caring about the outcome. Playing to win and being competitive is totally fine too. I will even add that some players are not coachable or certainly more difficult to coach. With coaching I mean helping a player, partnership or team utilize their current skills and resources to be more effective and successful. As stated, not all coaches are equal in perspective and abilities. If you are fortunate to have a pro/coach/teacher you like or who works for you, use them to help develop your potential. We all have room for improvement if we are willing to obtain it.

As a captain or co-captain, recruiting fresh players makes sense especially if they are a good fit. If possible, be selective based on what your team needs and wants to accomplish. There is a good fit for all players, and you need to be patient to attract and find a good team or partnership for you. Being frustrated and unhappy with your team situation may be an opportunity to proactively move on and find a better fit for you. This is when your instructor or coach can assist you with team/ partnership options. Certain flex leagues allow you to play with the same partner, and you have more control when you play your matches. Also, participating in local round robins and clinics can help you find players you like and want to play with. If you have access to courts in your city or community you may be able to find players in your area, plug into an existing league or ladder, and organize your own league or activity. More online apps and tools are now available that provide another option to find courts, other players for practice or match play, and perhaps instructors in your area or a city you are visiting.

With your involvement in tennis and in particular league tennis, you position yourself to fully enjoy and benefit from the sport at any age and level. Your skills should improve, and you will obtain new friends and opportunities that can enhance your lifestyle. We all need to obtain regular exercise, laugh, offset stress, and have fun! Meeting new people and making new friendships is a bonus. If you can play league tennis, make it fun and make it work for you!

SMART DOUBLES

CHAPTER 12

TEACHING PROFESSIONALS AND COACHES: SMART DOUBLES® AFFILIATION

D oubles Leagues along with their participants are excellent sources of revenue and referrals for facilities and teaching pros. Also, they are an extremely important feature for a facility's unique personality, overall program quality and financial success. In other words, tennis facilities, both public and private, typically do and should add value to a city, community, or area. Tennis courts alone *resting in peace* without programming do not serve the community well or the growth of tennis at large. In addition, each tennis facility or club is managed differently depending on the type of facility and the area. Also, each facility comes with its unique staff and management. In other words, some facilities and clubs are well managed and do a good job serving up a variety of quality tennis opportunities for their members or community, and some are not well managed that do an average to poor job. Just like I have seen a lot of dumb doubles, I have seen poorly managed facilities that underperform and underserve their marketplace.

As tennis teaching/coaching professionals in the tennis industry at large, we serve as advisors and leaders, and must care enough about our sport to share best practices that create more fun, excitement, benefits and success for our players and programs. I have enjoyed helping others learn and grow their skills so they can experience the fun and benefits connected to tennis. Seeing and hearing about how my students used their skills in real play is especially exciting. How do we as instructors, coaches, managers, and owners systematically deliver more equipped doubles players to their biggest stage and opportunity for playing and enjoying recreational doubles? In other words, how do we help convert more noncore, infrequent, and occasional players to core players? As stated in an article, *Numbers Game* that was published in May of 2019 by the Tennis Industry Magazine that quoted the current Tennis Industry Association Executive Director, Jolyn de Boer, "core players buy nearly 90 percent of all tennis gear, lessons, and court time, and the more avid the player, the more they contribute to the overall tennis economy".

As you know, teaching and coaching are similar but different. Just like singles and doubles are uniquely different. A private lesson with one person is quite different compared to a small group lesson/clinic. As a teaching professional, it is important to "keep it simple" so that your students and players can process and apply easily important basic concepts. At the Colony Beach & Tennis Resort, we called this approach "Success Now". Also, there is a wide variety of instructors regarding their playing styles, playing experience, teaching experience and personalities. At times, there can be a difference in opinion, approach or conflict between instructors when conducting clinics together or separately with groups or teams. Realistically, our egos and old habits can get in the way at times related to being open to innovative ideas such as open stances, swinging volleys, and the semi-western and western grip. As you know, dynamic stretching is more effective and safer than static stretching. It seems old habits die hard.

How we deliver tennis instruction and coaching to individuals and groups is very personal. In this learning environment it takes courage and being open for both parties to give and receive. Simultaneously, both student and coach are in a learning mode. For example, what works for one student or most in a small group may or may not work for another. Also, some students are more visual, some tend to over think, and some are not good listeners especially to a lot of verbiage. Less is more and KISS (keep it simple sally) are helpful teaching aides. Knowing your audience and being willing and able to adjust is a learning process too.

I have authored this book to make it easier, less technical, and more FUN for recreational players to *effectively* and *efficiently* learn and implement Smart Doubles® with or without a coach/instructor. But preferably, with a teaching pro or coach. In this book, I have chosen not to provide superfluous information about my doubles playing background, matches and victories or the matches and victories of other high-level players. My purpose is simply to enable, equip, and empower a large population of recreational players with basic doubles concepts that can be easily understood and implemented in games and matches. As you can imagine, a significant percentage of recreational players are self-taught for various reasons. Also, with this book, I hope to make teaching/coaching *doubles strategy and positioning* more fun, exciting and effective for teaching professionals and coaches. With Smart Doubles®, I seek to promote a doubles language or lingo that is easy for the student to absorb, apply and communicate about their intent, purpose, performance, and experience on the court playing doubles. Lessons, clinics, drills, and live ball are all great activities with a teaching pro. But what happens without the pro in their regular fun games or league matches may be a bigger learning and reinforcing experience for the student because of a good performance or a poor performance. As a coach, I want to know more about their "center stage" experience such as: Did you place most of your volleys- **Short to Short**- or put them back in play- short to deep? Did you sit in NML or transition to the party? Did you do a good job keeping the ball away from the net guy-**Deep to Deep**? Did you follow the ball well today at net? How many **One and Done** or *Money Middle* shots did you hit today? How was your serve today? Did you commit to more high-percentage shots that work for you most of the time? Did you change your formations as needed? How was your communication with your partner? When a student says to me, "I can hear you in my head," I know she is focused and committed to playing Smart Doubles®.

If you are a tennis instructor, coach, certified teaching professional or facility manager, hopefully, you see and appreciate the purpose, benefit, and opportunity associated with the Smart Doubles® program. Hopefully, you see Smart Doubles® as a fun, effective way to enhance your program for both your existing players and your incoming players. By implementing and promoting Smart Doubles®, you can attract fresh players, grow your membership, enhance your doubles-oriented program and enthusiasm at your club or facility. Becoming a Smart Doubles® affiliate creates a positive partnership that allows you to legally use my registered trademark at your club or facility in concert with the Smart Doubles® program.

Through the Smart Doubles® website, I seek to build a value-added bridge between recreational doubles players, organized leagues, and a community of coaches/teaching professionals/ facilities who are enthusiastic about playing, teaching, coaching, and promoting Smart Doubles®.

In my Smart Doubles program®, I promote and use specific clinics numbered 1, 2 and 3 to attract, place and teach certain players at three general levels. In short, for example, 2.5-3.0 players need more emphasis on *Deep to Deep* consistency, serving, returning, and proper positioning for doubles play. Players at 3.5-4.0 may need more focus on *Short to Short*, *FTB*, anticipating lobs, teamwork, and communication. Players at 4.0 and up may need more emphasis on poaching, *Low You Go*, transition, first volleys, and controlling the net. Using and promoting three or more general clinic options for your Smart Doubles® program makes it feasible to reach more players and help your players improve their specific skills for success now at doubles play. These tiered clinics with 3-6 participants compared to single person privates or semi-privates are a terrific format to teach Smart Doubles®, and to better integrate and direct more players to teams, leagues, mixers, partnerships, and related doubles events.

As an active pro, I enjoy the Three and Me clinic that allows me to "play in" to provide good examples and situations. Lastly, Smart Doubles® inspired events such as supervised match play for teams and round robins organized and managed by a pro or team captain can help build quality teams, create quality clinics/lessons, and improve the overall quality of play, enthusiasm, and success among recreational players at your facility. If your facility, club, or courts are doubles oriented, it makes sense to work smart by teaching and promoting the language of Smart Doubles®. In my view, Smart Doubles® can be the vehicle to drive new, interested, and current players into a more enjoyable and active lifestyle. The Smart Doubles® program creates more simplicity, effectiveness, success, and harmony for my players and for me as a teaching pro/coach. It can do the same for you and your players. At Smartdoubles.com you can learn more about becoming a Smart Doubles® affiliate. Let's partner up and grow the game of doubles and make it fun!

CONCLUSION

I hope the implementation of Smart Doubles® by additional teaching professionals at additional facilities will make it easier for new, inactive, and current players to learn, improve, excel, enjoy, and benefit from tennis on a regular basis through the fun, social game of doubles. I believe Smart Doubles®, if promoted and implemented at your club, facility or community can do just that. Hopefully, as a current player, you have gained valuable tips, tools, tactics, and strategy from Smart Doubles® that you can implement to create more enjoyment and success for you now on the tennis court.

As tennis professionals, individually and collectively, we can grow tennis in our communities by making it more accessible, easier to learn and fun to play through Smart Doubles® clinics. At certain times of the year tennis is extremely popular on television because of several major tennis events. However, in your local community tennis may or may not be popular or accessible on a weekly or daily basis. A good start would be to find nearby courts to organize play or create a program. Access to programs and the enjoyment of tennis by a larger audience of players will be driven by our delivery methods. Daily, we can teach mostly private lessons-one person- or more clinics- 4-6 persons. We can conduct supervised match play or round robins on several courts with one or more coaches to be sure players and partnerships are playing Smart

Doubles®. In addition, now we can teach online to hundreds or thousands and even travel as an independent to the student's court or community to reach and teach more students. The more players and students we encourage, empower, and equip to play, the more players we can better direct, deliver and integrate into the fun, social and beneficial recreational tennis environment.

Only a small percentage of players will reach an elite/ advanced level of skills to play varsity collegiate tennis or play professionally. For example, according to the ITF's 2021 Participation Report, there were 7,275 ranked juniors by the ITF, and 3,619 ATP and WTA ranked players or professionals.[7] Therefore, there will always be a larger population of junior and adult recreational players below 5.0 (NTRP) seeking casual to formal opportunities to enjoy and benefit from the sport. In junior programs not all kids can or want to excel at tennis. It is okay for them just to enjoy the game for fun, exercise, activity, and comradery. At some point juniors will become adults and can enjoy recreational tennis for a lifetime as well. *In my view, doubles is the best game that provides more benefits and enjoyment for more people globally and locally.* In addition, there is medical research that shows a lifestyle of regular tennis is beneficial for your heart and longevity. [5] Hopefully, for you, Smart Doubles® will become a language of love for your favorite game, sport, and activity.

During the Covid Pandemic, I decided to author this book to reach as many people as possible with my Smart Doubles® program. Enabling more recreational players from levels 2.5 -

4.5 NTRP to participate in doubles properly, intelligently, and confidently is a win-win for players, league organizations and teams, facilities, and our profession of teaching and coaching. It seems that most of us are willing to pay a premium for smart phones, smart TVs, and smart watches. Let's play, enjoy, promote, and teach Smart Doubles®!

ACKNOWLEDGEMENTS

I want to thank my lovely wife, Brenda, for her encouragement to finish and publish this book. I could not and would not have committed to authoring my first book without your support. Thank you for reading, rereading, and assisting me with editing. I am so blessed to have you as my partner for life on and off the court. Love You! Thanks Babe!

Also, I want to thank Eli, my Book Consultant and Stacey, my Editor for their professional contributions to my book. I appreciate your expertise and patience. I am grateful for all my students and tennis colleagues in Atlanta, Georgia, and in Sarasota/Longboat Key, Florida for the opportunity to learn from you and work with you. I am especially grateful for my first coach, friend, and unexpected mentor, Mr. Steve Christian whom I timely met at 12 years of age one summer day while hitting against the wall at Dunbar Community Center in Little Rock, Arkansas.

Finally, I am extremely grateful for the opportunity to play tennis and share tennis with others over several decades as a teaching professional.

REFERENCES

1. ALTA league. (2023). *Atlanta Lawn Tennis Association.* www.altatennis.org

2. Bedingfield, S. (2015). Doubles Tips and Tactics: A Tennis Guide for Women.

3. Francesconi, P. (2019 May). Numbers Game. Tennis Industry Magazine. Industry research.pdf (tennisindustrymag.com)

4. Green, M. R. (Director). (2021). *King Richard* [Film] Westbrook Studios.

5. Harr, S. (2023 January 17). America's War Against Heart Disease. AARP. Fighting Heart Disease in the United States (aarp.org)

6. International Tennis Federation. (2023). *Approved Balls.* ITFTennis.com/approved balls

7. International Tennis Federation. (2021). *International Tennis Federation's Global Tennis Report.* ITF - ITF Global Tennis Report 2021 (uberflip.com)

8. Schnohr, P., O'Keefe, J. H., Holtermann, A., Lavie, C. J., Lange, P., Jensen, G. B., & Marott, J. L. (2018). Various Leisure-Time Physical Activities Associated with Widely Divergent Life Expectancies: The Copenhagen City Heart Study. *Mayo Clinic Proceedings, 93*(12), 1775–1785. https://doi.org/10.1016/j.mayocp.2018.06.025

9. Sprecher, S. H. (2019, September 1). Tennis: A Game Changer in Park Revitalization. *Parks and Recreation.* Tennis: A Game Changer in Park Revitalization | Feature | Parks and Recreation Magazine | NRPA

10. T2Tennis. (2021). The flexible way to play. www.T2Tennis.com

11. (2021, September/October). *2021 TIA Tennis Industry Participation Report.* industry-research.pdf (tennisindustrymag.com)

12. Ultimate Tennis. (2023). www.ultimatetennis.com

13. Universal Tennis. (2022). www.universaltennis.com

14. USTA. (2023). *Leagues.* USTA League

ABOUT THE AUTHOR

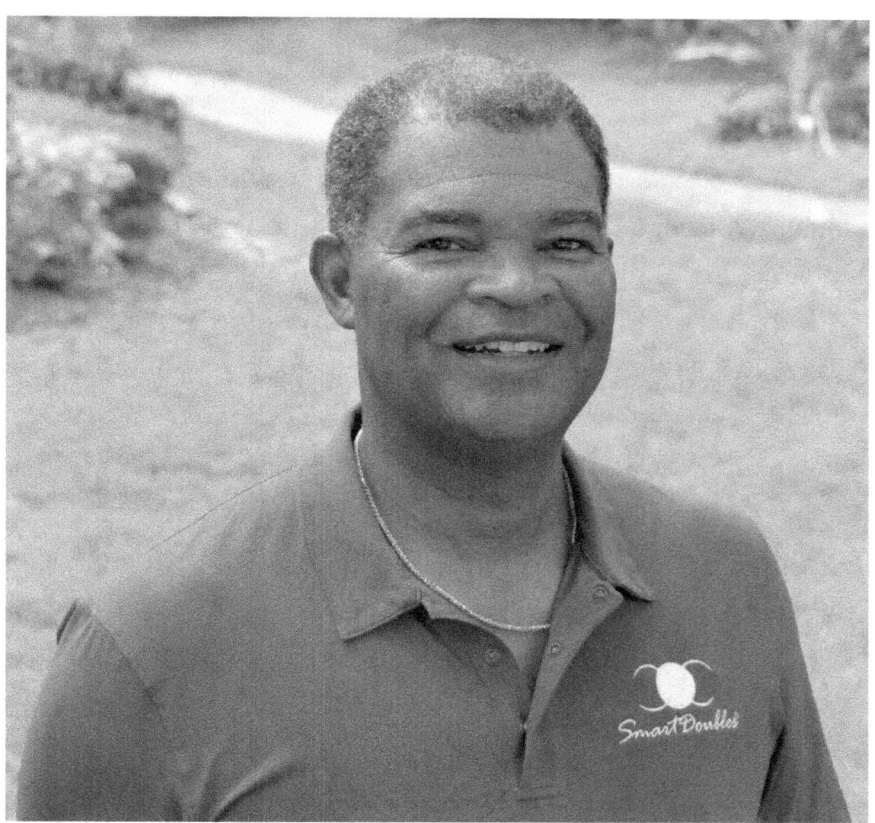

Ron Shields, author, and founder of Smart Doubles® grew up in Little Rock, Arkansas. In the city of Little Rock, he was informally introduced to tennis around the age of eight at the nearby, historic Central High school. Central was within biking or walking distance from his childhood home. Without access to public sector or private club junior programming and consistent private lessons, he managed to become a top ten ranked junior in his home state of Arkansas. Upon beginning high school at Hall High in the fall of 1976, Ron joined the varsity tennis team and played all three years on an extremely competitive state championship level team.

In the pursuit of becoming a collegiate and playing professional, he accepted a full tennis scholarship to Texas Southern University in Houston, Texas. After completing his first year at TSU in 1981, he transferred to the University of Arkansas at Little Rock as a walk-on for tennis. This relocation allowed him to be closer to his mother who previously suffered from a stroke. His teaching career officially began in 1983 at the Little Rock Racquet Club while attending UALR. In 1986, he graduated from the University of Arkansas at Little Rock with a BBA in Marketing. After working as an assistant teaching instructor from 1983-1989 at the Little Rock Racquet Club, Ron became a certified teaching professional by the U.S.P.T.A in 1992. In 1993, Ron relocated to Atlanta, Georgia.

During his first year in Atlanta, he coached and trained nationally and regionally ranked juniors at the Norman Wilkerson Academy at Sugar Creek Tennis Center and the Ralston Gorman Academy in various suburban locations. In Atlanta, from the spring of 1993 to the summer of 2004, he worked as a head pro/director at various facilities including Sugar Creek Tennis Center, Tucker Racquet Club, Bitsy Grant and Piedmont Park, and the Marcus Jewish Community Center.

Also, Ron worked as an independent teaching professional in the northern suburbs of Atlanta. As a competitive player, he thoroughly enjoyed playing league doubles at AA1 and AA2 levels and USTA mixed doubles among other teaching pros, former collegiate players, and touring pros. Ron was regularly active as a player and coach in the #1 league tennis metropolitan area in the USA and perhaps the world where he coached many ALTA and USTA league teams per season at all levels.

In the summer of 2004, Ron relocated to Bradenton, Florida. In the fall of 2004, he accepted an opportunity to work as a staff professional at the #1 ranked Colony Beach & Tennis Resort on Longboat Key, Florida. After the unfortunate first closing of the historic Colony in 2009 followed by the final closing in 2010, Ron began teaching at the Longboat Key Club & Resort which later became a top ten tennis resort in the world. He has enjoyed teaching residents, club members and seasonal tourists on Longboat Key since 2004. Ron is very passionate and gifted at teaching/coaching doubles strategy and positioning clinics now known as Smart Doubles®. He has enjoyed an extensive and successful teaching career in the public, private, residential and hospitality sectors for 30 plus years. In addition, he became a Certified Health Coach in 2011 with a passion for healthy living and nutrition.

In 2020, during the Covid- 19 pandemic, Ron made a commitment to writing and publishing his Smart Doubles® program. Also, he began writing a more personal book about his unique journey that featured tennis and personal growth.

This journey was inspired by certain loving, caring, and supportive people who had a major impact on his life and career. In his next book to follow Smart Doubles®, he will share humbling and unique details about how his love for tennis and related relationships have greatly enriched his life. In 2021, Ron and Brenda launched a Tennis For Fun affiliate program (tennisforfun.org) in partnership with Special Olympics in Sarasota. This program provides free weekly clinics to athletes with special needs and the opportunity to compete with other athletes at regional and state Special Olympics sponsored events.

In June of 2023, Ron was awarded the Regional USPTA Professional of the year award at Florida's USPTA Division Conference in Orlando. He was recognized for his dedication and involvement in the Tennis For Fun program, and his long-term professional affiliation with the USPTA.

Ron resides on Longboat Key, Florida with his lovely wife Brenda, and their spunky Biewer Terrier, Ashe.

OTHER PRODUCTS & SERVICES FROM SMART DOUBLES®

Instead of just writing a book, I decided to reinforce the Smart Doubles® program with certain merchandise such as hats, visors, shoe bags and towels that can only be purchased individually or in bundles at my web site. In addition, I will create and maintain promotional relationships with recreational doubles leagues and professional affiliations with specific clubs, facilities, and resorts.

Books purchased from my site will be autographed and shipped to buyers in the USA and Canada. Also, books will be available for purchase at other major online bookstores and select retailers.

Please contact me
regarding merchandise or
to inquire about a professional affiliation at:
www.SmartDoubles.com

In health,
Ron Shields | Smart Doubles LLC

www.ingramcontent.com/pod-product-compliance
Lightning Source LLC
Chambersburg PA
CBHW060531130626
46553CB00002B/706